THE PAPERLESS HOSPITAL

Healthcare in a Digital Age

THE PAPERLESS HOSPITAL

Healthcare in a Digital Age

Russell C. Coile, Jr.

Health Administration Press
ACHE Management Series

HIMSS

Your board, staff, or clients may also benefit from this book's insight. For more information on quantity discounts, contact the Health Administration Press Marketing Manager at (312) 424-9470.

05 04 03 02 01   5 4 3 2 1

Library of Congress Cataloging-in-Publication Data

Coile, Russell C.
    The paperless hospital : healthcare in a digital age / by Russell C. Coile, Jr.
      p. cm.
    Includes bibliographical references.
    ISBN 1-56793-162-6 (alk. paper)
        1. Hospitals—Administration. 2. Computer networks. 3. Internet. I. Title.
    [DNLM: 1. Delivery of Health Care—organization & administration. 2. Computer Communication Networks. 3. Hospital Administration—trends. 4. Internet.
    W 84.1 C679p 2001]

    RA971.23 .C65 2001
    362.1'1'068—dc21

                                                              2001039442

The paper used in this publication meets the minimum requirements of American National Standard for Information Sciences—Permanence of Paper for Printed Library Materials, ANSI Z39.48-1984. ∞ ™

Acquisitions manager: Audrey Kaufman; Project manager: Joyce Sherman; Text and cover design: Matt Avery

Health Administration Press
A division of the Foundation of the American
    College of Healthcare Executives
1 North Franklin Street, Suite 1700
Chicago, IL 60606-3491
(312) 424-2800

Healthcare Information and
    Management Systems Society
230 East Ohio Street
Suite 500
Chicago, IL 60611-3269

A project like this takes me away from my family more than I like to be reminded. I want to dedicate this book to my family, Nancy, Amanda, and Ariel, who will live in the digital future.

Table of Contents

Foreword to The Paperless Hospital: Healthcare in a Digital Age

LIKE ANY REVOLUTION, the digital transformation of healthcare began almost imperceptibly many years ago. I witnessed one of its earliest events without having any special awareness of what was to come. The 400-bed hospital where I worked as a photographer installed its first computer in the late 1960s, and I was asked to take pictures for the press release announcing the hospital's entry into the new world of electronic data processing. The computing machine was more noteworthy for its size than for its function. I remember the hospital's public relations director asking me to take pictures to showcase the half-dozen new, refrigerator-sized boxes that filled an air-conditioned room in the basement.

The automation of financial record keeping was not the big story. The important message was that our hospital's computer was literally bigger than the neighboring hospital's computer. A few employees joked about being "replaced by a button," but if anything was presumably foreshadowed by our new data processor, it was that even bigger machines were coming. Indeed, the president of International Business Machines (IBM) predicted at the time that the world would soon be run by a handful of very big supercomputers. As best I can remember, all the attention was focused on computers as business machines. They were going to make traditional business more efficient, providing better ways to do the same old things. Conventional wisdom circa 1970 did not dictate that computers would redefine the very foundations of business. And absolutely no one thought that the telecommunications industry would ever become a force of change.

Now, only three decades later, big mainframes have all but disappeared. Computer science and telecommunications are together creating a new realm of possibilities out of millions of small machines that sit on our desks, rest in our laps, or hang from our belts. The networked computer has put incredible power in the hands of end users, allowing anyone with basic applications skills to redesign a work process, get previously protected information, develop a new product, or organize special interest groups. Just as the development of moveable type transformed the world by making the Bible available to the masses, the development of modern telecomputing is creating a Reformation in many domains—including healthcare.

This book is an excellent overview of coming changes to the extent they can be foreseen by experts in the field. Russ Coile has done a superb job of collecting the perspectives of a wide variety of commentators, distilling their observations into common themes, and providing a wealth of practical hints for anyone who wants to understand or influence the evolution of healthcare in the first decade of the twenty-first century. Much has been said on these general themes over the past few years, and this book is an excellent compendium of that information. It is a worthy document from one of the country's best-known health futurists.

Russ himself would be the first to admit that the future is going to be full of surprises, especially in such a high-tech area as healthcare. Nevertheless, the inherent uncertainty of making predictions is not a valid reason for ignoring the many fascinating observations made in the coming pages. Many of the scenarios are likely to come true, and even those that do not materialize as envisioned today may provide the creative spark for visionaries who find even better ways to maximize the benefits of the digital transformation. This book conveys a sense of excitement about the future, and that is a message much needed in healthcare today.

Russ Coile's book also dispels an unfortunate perception that the digital transformation of healthcare is a myth because so many dot-com companies failed over the past year. Many companies that were Wall Street's dreams in 2000 are investors' nightmares in 2001, but the problem is not a result of flawed technology. Many high-tech healthcare companies lost their luster because they did not have a business plan or a competent management team, and many investors lost their money because they were seduced by the mass hysteria of irrational expectations. Chalk the failures up to incompetence and greed.

Instead, focus on the possibilities for digital transformation. I spend most of my professional life studying how networked computers are changing healthcare, and I do not see any evidence that the revolution has failed. I do not even think that progress has been perceptibly slowed by the debacle in the financial markets. Thousands of healthcare leaders, including a remarkable number of visionary physicians and other experienced clinicians, are still going to work every day to do the research and development that will revolutionize medicine. Private and public capital is still flowing into this field, and lots of companies are following reasoned, results-oriented business plans. The hype may be gone, but the promise is not. Healthcare in 2010 will not look much like healthcare in 2001. This book is a great guide for anyone who wants to know why, or—better yet—anyone who wants to help bring about the changes.

Jeff Bauer
Hillrose, Colorado
July 2001

Preface: Healthcare Executives Straddle the "Digital Divide" [1]

"THERE ARE PERHAPS few industries that have more to gain from the Internet revolution than medicine ... [but doctors and] hospitals are real laggards when it comes to the Internet. What e-health has to be used for is to transform the whole process of delivering care."

—*Russell Ricci, M.D. (Steinhauer 2000)*

The digital transformation of healthcare is a work in process, and "We are not there yet," declares Anne Seger, M.D., Medical Director of System Integration for University of Massachusetts Memorial Hospital in Boston (Steinhauer 2000, p. E1). The visionaries, entrepreneurs, and venture capitalists are gone after the collapse of the "e-health" bubble. Now the real work begins, transforming 5,000 hospitals and 20,000 medical groups into electronically integrated healthcare systems that manage patients with "seamless" care. The health system of tomorrow may never be entirely "paperless," but progress is being made despite the legendary reluctance of physicians to accept changes in the way they practice medicine. Rapid advancements in biotechnology and medical research, increasingly curious patients who shop the World Wide Web for medical information, and pressures from managed care companies to contain costs and speed treatments are just the central components driving the e-health scenario.

As a senior consultant for Superior Consultant Corporation, Inc., a national consulting firm based in Southfield, Michigan that specializes in digital business solutions for the health field, I see the electronic transformation of healthcare first hand. Despite reluctance to embrace the "e"-revolution, many hospitals and medical groups are employing the Internet and information technology to improve their customer interface as well as to reduce business costs. Healthcare executives must straddle the digital divide between hospital managers and doctors who have embraced information technology, versus the "show-me-the-data" skeptics among physicians and administrators who will be the last to use a computer in the executive suite or medical office.

The shocking collapse of many Internet companies in 2000 has thrown a wet blanket on the e-health industry. Venture capital has dried up in the sector, and financial woes have battered firms such as drkoop .com, PlanetRx, and WebMD. *A caution as you read this book:* Estimates of e-health revenues and growth should be taken with a grain of salt. Shattuck Hammond Partners, a respected Wall Street firm, recently issued a report that compares the e-health mania of 1999 and early 2000 with the "tulipmania," a boom-and-bust episode that swept The Netherlands and Europe in the seventeenth century (Dickey 2000). A more realistic appraisal of e-health's future is emerging, in which information technology and Internet-based connectivity are integrated into virtually every aspect of healthcare over the next five to ten years.

THE BUSINESS CASE FOR E-HEALTH

The business case for e-health is now being demonstrated from the critical care unit to the loading dock. Electronic solutions can reduce costs by improving physician productivity, reducing clerical and administrative expenses, automating price shopping and ordering to cut supply and pharmaceutical expenditures, and treating patients more cost-efficiently. Sharing data on the Internet is a better, faster, cheaper solution. But e-health strategy gets complicated when hospitals and medical groups try to determine how to integrate their legacy information systems and software with the new Internet applications. Many e-vendors offer "plug-and-play" ease of installation and use, but few applications hold up to the realities of harried staffers, techno-skeptical physicians, and limited capital due to fiscal hits from managed care and the Balanced Budget Act.

In the new millennium, the Internet will become the "hub of healthcare," predicts John Morrisey, information editor for *Modern Healthcare* (Morrisey 1999). The rapid growth of Web-based connectivity is a strong "push" factor for deployment of e-solutions in healthcare. Web-based systems are far easier and less expensive to acquire, maintain, and service than client-server or mainframe-based systems.

Many chief information officers (CIOs) believe that the Internet makes provider organizations an offer they cannot refuse—lower costs, widespread access, and interface engines for in-place hardware and software. Within this decade, Web technology will eventually replace most traditional models (Kilbridge 2000). Already, the healthcare market is seeing a consolidation of legacy information technology providers with newer Intranet companies to offer integrated e-technology solutions. E-health experts at Superior Consultant project savings in a number of areas, such as (Coile 2000):

- supply-chain management strategies, which give purchasers the lowest-cost access to all products, saving 10 to 15 percent on every purchase;
- e–managed care connections, which reduce the cost of verifying insurance eligibility from $32 per patient to $.060, and electronic authorization of treatment, which slashes provider back-office expenses from $16 per case to $1.60;
- Internet-connected care management programs, which speed lab results to physicians, provide computer-based care plans on admission, and lower length of stay by 0.5 to 1.0 days, cutting cost-per-case by $400 to $1,000 for each patient;
- "e-cash" systems, which accelerate electronic claims and payments, reducing days-in-receivables, and pumping millions of dollars into hospital cash flows;

- outsourcing information systems, which saves 10 to 15 percent per year, and sale-leaseback of information technology, which can free up millions of dollars of capital for alternative investments or improved profitability; and
- creation of a hospital or health system intranet for physicians, which reduces information systems and information technology operating and capital investment expenses for doctors, and browser-facilitated access to real-time data on their patients, which enhances physician loyalty, resulting in 10 to 15 percent improvement in physician referrals.

The Internet's impact on the doctor-patient relationship is at the heart of the digital transformation scenario, which is shifting power from practitioner to patient (Bauer and Coile 2000). Consumers now have unprecedented access to health information from thousands of health-oriented web sites. Consumers can use online databases to select a doctor according to their preferences, join chat rooms and discussion groups, or purchase prescriptions and other medical supplies from a wide variety of online retailers. The e-frontier is still developing, so consumers will continue to have even more opportunities to perform functions that were traditionally managed by doctors.

NEW TECHNOLOGY

Technological developments will hasten the digital transformation of healthcare. Within the next two to five years, a number of advances in telecommunications and Internet infrastructure can be expected (Bauer 1999).

- The Internet backbone is being redesigned by a consortium of public and private organizations, and the second general Net will be widely available in the twenty-first century. It will be faster and more secure, and it will have much greater capabilities to handle multimedia traffic, such as that driven by telephony, video, and massive databases.

- The "last mile" problem of linking low-bandwith channels, such as copper wire, to the Web's high-speed backbone, fiber-optic cable, will gradually be solved as consumers get direct access to broadband services from their homes and offices via cable and wireless networks.
- The look and feel of the Web will be enhanced and its functionality improved by a new approach to programming. Hypertext markup language (HTML), the software that is currently used for most Web pages, effectively limits the Web to static images. The new language, extensible markup language (XML), in addition to supporting a much richer slice of virtual reality, will solve many problems associated with hardware and software incompatibility.
- Better computer operating systems and more powerful search engines are expected to be widely distributed in the near future. Users will be able to go directly to desired information faster than ever before. The new systems will eliminate many of the inefficiencies that have hindered use of the Web until now.
- Wireless technology will make the concept of "being wired" obsolete. The rapid deployment of wireless-enabled, hand-held personal digital assistant–type devices will transform telecommunications. In medical applications, wireless technology will finally cut the cord of dependence on paper records, providing doctors and nurses with a lightweight, portable electronic medical record that will be universally accessible across a medical unit or metropolitan area.

E-ORGANIZATION CULTURE

The ultimate barriers and enablers of the digital transformation are not technical—they are cultural. When healthcare executives, physicians, nurses, health plans, suppliers, and patients embrace e-technology, the information revolution will have finally arrived. A digital divide still exists between e-users and e-skeptics, and healthcare is traditionally slow to adopt new technology. Most healthcare executives prefer to buy "second-generation" technology, and only 25 to 35 percent of physicians use the Internet for patient care.

Patients are providing the momentum for healthcare's digital transformation. Over 100 million Americans have Internet access now, and more than half of them—52 million in 2000—sought health information and advice on the Web. Availability of low-cost information technology and Internet access is driving a fundamental realignment of the patient-provider relationship. Dr. George Whitesides of Harvard University warns that "the conventional medical system could lose control ... to groups of patients, people who are ill, talking to one another and convincing themselves that the alternatives lie elsewhere than in the clinical system" (Mitka 1999). Although that possibility is remote, it could happen if health professionals and delivery systems try to prevent or control consumer empowerment. Providers must recognize that the information genie is out of the bottle. The digital transformation of healthcare will reinvent the practice of medicine and the management of health organizations in the twenty-first century.

OUTLINE OF THE BOOK

Read this book like you would survey a banquet table. Search for what interests you, and read those chapters first, and in more detail. Skim other chapters that are less critical to your immediate needs. Come back to study additional content areas in the days and months ahead, as the e-revolution becomes more widespread and influential in healthcare organizations. Pass the book along to colleagues and coworkers, as e-health extends its reach across hospitals, physician offices, health plans, and the many community settings where healthcare is provided.

A brief introduction to each chapter is outlined below. You will find that strategic implications are projected at the conclusion of each chapter.

Chapter 1—Introduction: The Digital Transformation of Healthcare

Utilizing e-health strategies will expand exponentially in the next five years, as America's healthcare executives shift to applying IS and IT to the fundamental business and clinical processes of the healthcare enterprise.

Chapter 2—Cyber-Health: Transforming Legacy Systems into Enterprise Application Infrastructures

Somewhere between the high promise of information technology and the all-too-real performance limitations of today's information systems, every American hospital, medical group, and health system is struggling to upgrade its IS and IT infrastructure to meet the demands of twenty-first-century healthcare.

Chapter 3—Report Cards: Competing in a Consumer-Driven Marketplace

The Internet is a growing source of report card information for "med-retrievers," the online health shoppers who are looking for the best doctors, treatments, and hospitals available. Employers are also interested in steering their employees to providers with the best outcomes and lowest error rates.

Chapter 4—Connecting Businesses

Migrating many of healthcare's business processes to the Internet offers great promise. Better business solutions, lower prices, and customized processes and products are all possible.

Chapter 5—E-Solutions: Harnessing the Internet for Business Improvement

E-solutions will provide new strategies to achieve both cost and revenue goals and create new relationships with patients, physicians, suppliers, health plans, and government agencies.

Chapter 6—Web Strategies: The Internet and Customer Relationship Management

The availability of health information on the Web is empowering consumers and fundamentally affecting the patient-physician relationship.

"Health-seekers" are a new category of Internet users who are searching online for disease-specific information, health advice, and guidance in selecting providers.

Chapter 7—Outsourcing: A Better, Faster, Cheaper Solution for Technology Management

Healthcare providers are utilizing outsourcing strategies to manage many noncore functions, such as web site maintenance, managing off-site data warehouses, and building and maintaining information networks with physicians. Outsourcing also offers healthcare providers the opportunity to acquire and distribute knowledge without the time and cost of producing that knowledge internally, such as Web content, consumer health information, and disease management.

Chapter 8—Call Centers: Managing Demand to Manage Care

Medicine's "virtual practice" era is rapidly arriving. Imagine primary care providers and specialists only seeing patients in their offices when absolutely necessary, with nurse and patient monitoring being conducted the rest of the time from the "electronic physician office," the call center.

Chapter 9—Telemedicine: A New Foundation for Healthcare Delivery

Web-based telemedicine applications promise lower costs, almost universal access, and multimodal capability to transmit a variety of data and images. Costs for telemedicine systems are falling rapidly, and digital video technology is providing small, low-cost cameras for two-way Web-enabled telecommunication with real-time streaming video.

Chapter 10—Medical Errors and the Science of Care Management

Quality improvement is a business strategy. Case studies in error reduction and medication management suggest substantial savings of millions of dollars can be achieved in typical hospitals.

Chapter 11—HIPAA, Electronic Privacy, and Internet Transactions

Under provisions of the Health Insurance Portability and Accountability Act of 1996, federal rules were released in 2001 that require compliance within two years. The federal legislation has also become a major vehicle for protecting patient privacy and ensuring the security of electronic medical records. HIPAA will fix the lack of electronic standards for data interchange in healthcare that has hampered the widespread deployment of e-commerce.

Chapter 12—Managing Healthcare's E-Organizations

As the digital transformation occurs within the health sector, every hospital, medical group, health plan, and supplier must face the "e-culture challenge" to prepare themselves for the move to an e-based set of internal processes and external relationships.

Russell C. Coile, Jr.
Plano, Texas

NOTE

1. This foreword is based in part on the article by Russell C. Coile, Jr., "Physician Executives Straddle the 'Digital Divide'," which appeared in *Physician Executive*, 27 (2): 12–19, March/April 2001.

REFERENCES

Bauer, J. C. 1999. *Telemedicine and Reinvention of Healthcare: The Seventh Revolution in Medicine.* New York: McGraw-Hill.

Bauer, J. C., and R. C. Coile, Jr. 2000. "Should Physicians Be Paid for Online Care? E-Frontier Challenges Traditional Reimbursement." *Medical Crossfire* 2 (10): 1–3.

Coile, R. C., Jr. 2000. "E-Solutions: Harnessing the Internet for Performance Improvement in Healthcare Organizations." *Health Trends* 12 (1): 1–12.

Dickey, K. 2000. "eHealth rEvolution," pp. 1–26. New York: Hammond Shattuck Partners.

Kilbridge, P. M. 2000. "Urging Providers to Embrace the Web." *MD Computing* 17 (1): 13–18.

Mitka, M. 1999. "Futurists See Longer, Better Life in the Third Millennium." *Journal of the American Medical Association* 281 (18): 1686.

Morrisey, J. 1999. "Just A Click Away." *Modern Healthcare* 29 (39): 5–7.

Steinhauer, J. A. 2000. "Health Revolution in Baby Steps." *New York Times*, October 25, pp. E1, E10–11.

Acknowledgments

The Paperless Hospital is dedicated to my colleagues and clients at Superior Consultant, Inc., who have provided insights and real-world examples of the application of digital business solutions to the health field. I want to express my appreciation to Rich Helppie, founder and CEO; Ron Aprahamian, chairman; George Huntzinger, president; Steve Smith, COO; Richard Sorenson, CFO; Sue Synor, executive vice president; and Charles Bracken, executive vice president. I am grateful for the support and ideas from many colleagues across the Superior organization, including Ed Bloski, Tom Easterly, Jerry Davis, Katy Derezinski, Joel French, Deborah Freund, Steve Gray, Evelyn Grindstaff, Cynthia Hayward, Julie Heintz, Ann Keillor, Dan Riina, and Steve Rushing. Special thanks to my "Sage Group" colleagues, Paul Bushnell, Jeff Bauer, Rick Krohn, and Nate Kaufman, who provide insights from the market. I rely daily on support from my practice assistant Debbie Sullivan, who is an invaluable asset, given my travel and speaking schedules. My very special thanks to Gail Oren, corporate research librarian, and her successor, Susan Waters, for their knowledge and assistance throughout the project, and to Marilyn Krainen, editor, for her help and advice.

CHAPTER ONE

Introduction: The Digital Transformation of Healthcare

KEY CONCEPTS: *B2B and B2C • Information economy • Adoption of technology • P2P • Telemedicine • Internet strategies*

INTRODUCTION: The arrival of the Internet offers the opportunity to fundamentally reinvent medicine and healthcare delivery. The "e-health" era is nothing less than the digital transformation of the practice of medicine as well as the business side of the health industry. Healthcare is only now arriving in the "information economy," and the Internet is the next frontier of healthcare. Healthcare consumers are flooding into cyberspace, and an Internet-based industry of health information providers is springing up to serve them. Internet technology may rank with antibiotics, genetics, and computers as among the most important changes for medical care delivery. Utilizing e-health strategies will expand exponentially in the next five years, as America's healthcare executives shift to applying information systems and information technology (IS and IT) to the fundamental business and clinical processes of the healthcare enterprise. Internet-savvy physician executives will provide a bridge between medicine and management in the adoption of e-health technology.

"THE eHEALTH SECTOR has tremendous potential for growth that we believe will eventually be realized. But in our view, the companies in the sector will generate value incrementally. In the short term, we will witness an eHealth evolution, not revolution. But over time, we are certain that the evolution of eHealth companies will, in sum, revolutionize the healthcare industry."

—*Shattuck Hammond Partners (2000, p. 1)*

The arrival of the Internet offers the opportunity to fundamentally reinvent medicine and healthcare delivery. The "e-health" era is nothing less than the digital transformation of the practice of medicine and of the business aspects of the health industry (Coile 2000). Healthcare is only now arriving in the information economy. Andrew Grove, chairman of Intel, predicts that "just as Email and the Internet have created an 'X-factor' that has stimulated the U.S. economy through increased productivity and efficiency, it is time for an 'X-factor' in healthcare, where Internet technology is used to keep costs in check while deepening [patient-provider] relationships through increased communication and care" (Ukens 1998).

The Internet's impact on the health field will be fundamental and sweeping, linking millions of providers, services, and settings into a seamless web of care. Consumers seeking health advice may scan the relevant medical literature in seconds and update their personal electronic medical records from their latest encounters with the health system. Healthcare will be a global industry, with patients seeking and finding the best-of-the-best medical practitioners and clinical centers of excellence with the aid of Internet-based "report cards" such as those provided by Healthgrades.com.

BEYOND E-HEALTH MANIA

Despite this optimistic outlook for the long term, the "e-health mania" of 1999–2000 has badly shaken the confidence of healthcare providers in their electronic strategies. The bottomless appetite of investors in e-based companies hit a wall in March 2000. Wall Street values for e-health companies shrank below 75 percent of their one-time highs, and companies like Healthgate.com have been delisted by NASDAQ because their share prices fell below minimum capital requirements.

Wall Street analysts at Shattuck Hammond Partners characterize the bruising fall of e-health companies as a "riches to rags" story (Shattuck Hammond 2000). The *Wall Street Journal* recently noted in one headline that "e-business booster Mary Meeker becomes e-lusive," commenting on the declining visibility of one of Wall Street's most prominent proponents of technology stocks who dropped out of the limelight since Internet stocks plummeted (Smith 2001).

Analysts attribute the rapid collapse of the e-health sector to (1) the slow pace of healthcare providers to adopt new technology, which limited market size and held down revenue growth of electronic enterprises; (2) frenzied capital flows into "e-anything," including many unproven concepts; and (3) willingness of investors to drive up the prices of e-based companies with little revenue and no clear path to achieve profitability. In the aftermath, a tremendous shakeout is occurring, with Internet-based companies downsizing or exiting. A new phase is now appearing—"bricks and clicks"—in which companies with existing non-Internet businesses are now deploying Web strategies and inventing new Internet companies. Examples include group purchasing, health insurance, and third-party intermediaries.

In the long term, the prospects for e-health are promising. The Internet and information technologies have radically reshaped other sectors of the economy, such as banking, airlines, and retail shopping. The use of the Internet to support true electronic commerce is accelerating in most industries, while the health industry and managed care seem to be stuck in first gear (Schaich 1999). That is changing rapidly, as the health industry is targeted by a wave of "dot-com" companies, such as drkoop.com, WebMD, HealthCentral, PlanetRx, and Health-Insurance.com. Wall Street experts tell investors to focus on the "three Cs"—connectivity, content, and commerce (Readerman 1999).

THE FRONTIER OF ELECTRONIC HEALTHCARE

The Internet is the next frontier of healthcare. Healthcare consumers are flooding into cyberspace, and an Internet-based industry of health information providers is springing up to serve them. A recent Harris Poll reported that in 1999, 70 million (74 percent) of the estimated 97

Figure 1.1: Online Health Content Used by Consumers

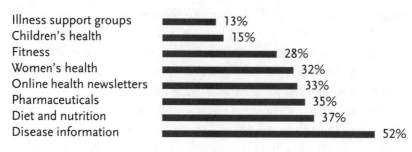

Illness support groups — 13%
Children's health — 15%
Fitness — 28%
Women's health — 32%
Online health newsletters — 33%
Pharmaceuticals — 35%
Diet and nutrition — 37%
Disease information — 52%

Source: Cyber Dialogue, cited in Marhula (1999, p. 14).

million people online have visited one or more of the Web's 20,000 health-related sites for medical information (Hochstadt and Lewis 1999). By 2005, the United States will have reached the end of its first digital decade, and 67 percent of the population will have Internet access, predicts Forrester Research (Business Wire 2001). Seniors are the latest population group to join the Internet revolution; call them the "wired retired." Older Americans are firing up personal computers and logging on to the Internet to arrange travel, manage their investments, e-mail their grandchildren, and seek health information. According to a recent survey, 21.3 percent of Medicare recipients had Internet access last year, up from 6.8 percent in 1997 (Wired Watch 2000). In response, the federal government has upgraded its web site, www.medicare.gov, expanding its online information on Medicare benefits, health plan options, and nursing home data.

Some consumers are turning to their local hospitals or health plans for health information, but many are employing the Web to search on a global basis for the latest medical research or evaluated treatment data (see Figure 1.1). Business-to-consumer (B2C) electronic commerce is an emerging healthcare market for drug refills, durable medical equipment, and alternative medicines. Prescription refills are one of the high-volume transactions that could be delivered at a very low cost. Some 25 percent of Internet users who go online for health information report interest in purchasing prescription drugs online. In response, pharmaceutical firms are projected to spend $11 billion on direct-to-consumer online advertising by 2005 (Marhula 1999). An estimated 60 percent of consumers using health web sites have purchased other products online.

Today's rapidly rising Web traffic on health sites is only the beginning. A recent study by Northwestern University and KPMG in Chicago affirms that baby boomers are the quintessential generation to demand what they want, fueled by Internet-available medical information (Howgill 1998). Healthcare providers with well-developed web sites, like Houston, Texas's MD Anderson and the Mayo Clinic in Rochester, Minnesota, will reinforce their brand identity and gain customer loyalty by providing easy Internet access to detailed health information. Many other hospitals and health systems are just starting to focus resources on Web-enabled electronic commerce and business applications such as marketing, physician directories, and employee recruitment, according to national data from the Health Information Management Systems Society (HIMSS).

B2B REINVENTS TRANSACTIONS AND COMMERCE

Although B2C Internet solutions are attracting millions of consumer "eyeballs," the real opportunity for the Internet is B2B, or business-to-business, commerce. Healthcare is a high-transaction business: an estimated 15 percent of all data transmissions in the United States are related to healthcare (Hochstadt and Lewis 1999). A simple doctor visit can generate five transactions, and a more complex cardiac evaluation involves 23 transactions. These transaction costs can be lowered by using the Internet. Electronically verifying insurance eligibility could reduce the transaction cost from $5 per patient to $0.60 per patient, with an annual savings of $10,000 for a busy doctor seeing 500 clients each month. The next wave of e-enabled applications will focus on creating new customer channels, e-commerce, electronic engineering of core processes, and supply-chain management (see Figure 1.2).

An estimated 25 percent of the nation's $1.3 trillion health budget is considered to be excessive administrative costs or unnecessary medical treatments (Marhula 1999). That is a $300 million business target

Figure 1.2: Spectrum of Healthcare E-Commerce Applications on the Internet

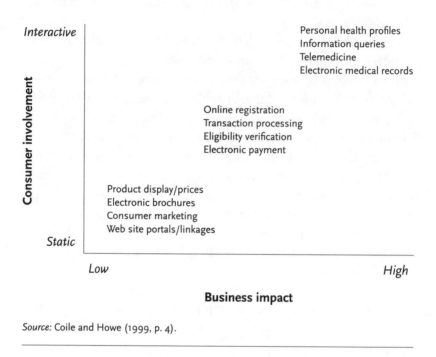

Source: Coile and Howe (1999, p. 4).

for the e-health economy, using Internet-enabled processes like disease management and supply-chain management. Only 6 percent of the healthcare industry uses the Internet for buying supplies today, compared to 25 percent of companies in other industries. In the digital marketplace, buying medical products on the Internet can reduce costs 5 to 15 percent or more, taking advantage of Web-enabled comparison shopping through companies like Medicalbuyer.com.

E-MEDICINE REINVENTS THE DOCTOR-PATIENT RELATIONSHIP

The Internet's global networks offer just what the health field has needed, a low-cost technology that bridges competing hardware and software to provide a seamless web of communications pathways. e-Medicine changes the patient-physician (P2P) relationship; in the process, it is reinventing medicine. Dot-com companies are moving rapidly to create new information sources and value-added transaction channels for healthcare providers, payers, purchasers, and suppliers.

Internet technology may rank with antibiotics, genetics, and computers as among the most important changes for medical care delivery, which futurist Jeffrey Bauer calls the "seventh revolution" in medicine (Bauer 1999). Some 20 to 60 percent of specialists' patients arrive at physicians' offices with articles from the Internet, including "cyberchondriacs," who may imagine they have the diseases they have double-clicked (Hochstadt and Lewis 1999).

America's 700,000 practicing physicians are logging on to the World Wide Web in record numbers. Market research data by the Healtheon Corporation show a 300 percent jump in regular Internet physician usage in the past two years (Healtheon 1999). In 1996, only 15 percent of U.S. physicians searched the Internet for clinical reasons. This figure climbed to 50 percent by mid-1997 and increased to 70 percent by the end of 1998. More recent data from the American Medical Association (AMA) find that 54 percent of physicians are using the Internet in their offices (AMA News 2001). Another 2001 survey by Deloitte Consulting and Cyber Dialogue found that 90 percent of 1,200 doctors had been online in the past 12 months, but only 55 percent used the Net daily, and only 24 percent used it for professional reasons.

In past surveys, doctors have cited "lack of time" as a primary reason for low use of the Internet for clinical information. But the latest report on physician usage of the Internet indicated that doctors now report that "lack of meaningful content and services" is the primary reason they do not rely on the Web more often for clinical purposes. These data suggest that issues of access and computer literacy are being overcome.

Sensing that doctors are ready to use the Web for business as well as clinical purposes, the AMA, in conjunction with other medical societies in the United States, has launched a new for-profit company, Medem, which operates web sites and provides services meant to compete with drkoop.com, Medscape, and WebMD. "We're trying to put the doctor back in the information loop," says Joe Sanders, Jr., M.D., executive director for the American Academy of Pediatrics, which is a cofounder of Medem (Carrns 1999). As for the commercial sites, Medscape may be gaining traction to advance its vision of electronic medicine, although the company lost over $300 million in 2000. The Hillsboro, Oregon–based medical electronics firm recently announced the sale of 5,000 handheld medical computers to General Motors (GM), which will distribute the computers to physicians in GM's health plan (*Modern Healthcare Daily* 2001). Drkoop and other content providers have established their place with consumers but are still searching for revenues and a sustainable business model (NASDAQ threatened to delist drkoop.com when its stock price fell below the exchange's minimum share price of $1 in February 2001).

CONSUMERS REINVENT HEALTHCARE ON THE INTERNET

Healthcare consumers are turning to the Web as an increasingly trustworthy source of health-related information, and consumer choices are rapidly expanding. Primary uses of the Web by health consumers in the future will include:

- disease-specific health information;
- directories of providers;
- health plan eligibility and benefits information;
- report card ratings of health plans and providers;
- patient support groups or chat rooms;
- online health advice and counseling;
- personal health risk assessment;
- order forms for books on health-related topics;
- search functions linked to medical literature for the latest medical advances;
- participation in clinical studies for pharmaceutical manufacturers;

- in-home monitoring of the chronically ill by disease management programs;
- prescription drug refills, over-the-counter remedies, and durable medical equipment;
- personalized electronic medical records; and
- monitoring of personal health improvement and fitness programs.

Internet access for patient self-scheduling is likely to be a popular service enhancement, allowing patients to scan their doctor's calendar and make appointments. The system can also provide Internet reminders electronically to patients 24 hours prior to appointments. The convenience of the Internet contrasts with today's appointment process, which often requires waiting long minutes on hold or following confusing voice mail instructions for help from a telephone-based central scheduling system.

Internet-based patient records will allow consumers to "own" their electronic medical records. Internet health information providers and some hospital web sites encourage consumers to register their health history and build a record of their health status over time. Universal patient identifiers such as social security numbers can provide an Internet address for future medical data from providers to be electronically compiled. The goal is to inform consumers, who then become empowered to monitor and manage their health improvement.

Patient support groups and chat rooms are creating "communities" of customers. Internet advocates believe that the ultimate use of the Internet in healthcare is to build learning communities of consumers and providers. More fundamentally, Internet-empowered consumers can take a leading role in promoting their own health and making effective use of their health plan and providers. Support groups of patients who share a diagnosis or treatment are among the most active healthcare users of the Internet. Patients share the latest medical literature and research findings and provide commentary on the efficacy of their treatments. Pharmaceutical companies and device makers are actively working with Web-based support groups, collaborating on research studies to obtain active participation in clinical trials, as well as facilitating the early distribution of newly approved drugs or devices. These Internet-linked communities of patients, providers, plans, and purchasers offer hope for collaboration and cost-efficiency in providing medical care in the new millennium.

TELEMEDICINE

What's next? E-medicine. Online health advice and telemedicine are overcoming regulatory and reimbursement barriers. With little regulation in place at this time, some healthcare providers are venturing into new territory—dispensing health advice online and even prescribing pharmaceuticals, for a fee. The practice is currently frowned upon by professional organizations and only quasi-legal under state medical licensure statutes, especially where the physician has never personally examined the patient. State-based regulators also express concern about health professionals doing business across state boundaries without state licenses. Online consultations for patients seeking Viagra are already available through web sites such as viagrapurchase .com, with 48-hour delivery of the drug, and regulators have initiated crackdowns on the practice in some states.

Physician skepticsm of Internet-based telemedicine is being overcome, and such practice could become widely utilized in the coming decade. At the Veterans Administration, chief information officer (cio) Robert Kolodner, m.d., states, "Much of our telemedical clinical activity could be translated to the Internet," based on the va's substantial telemedicine experiments in cross-country pathology and remote medical consultation (Baldwin 1998). Low-cost, Internet-based telemedicine will become a cost-effective method for remote diagnosis, patient information, case management and monitoring, and remote medical consultation. Donald Berwick, m.d., president of the Institute for Health Care Improvement in Boston, reports: "I met with 100 doctors the other night ... and they love it. But you should have heard the concerns they had," especially about inability to get paid for anything but a face-to-face visit (Kolata 2001).

VIRTUAL CHAINS OF PROVIDERS

Imagine a national network of the finest cardiac surgeons and cardiologists, or the nation's world-class cancer centers, all organized in a virtual network, contracted to the nation's largest health plans, and available at a mouse click. Ambitious efforts to link doctors and hospitals into national companies have failed in part due to the lack of a low-cost communications architecture that could integrate them into truly nationwide firms. The Internet offers an opportunity to restructure medicine and hospital care beyond regional or state boundaries.

The Internet is becoming an online catalog for choosing providers. Colorado-based HealthGrades.com provides limited online directory information on 600,000 physicians now (HealthGrades does not yet rate physicians with its "five-star" ranking system as it does for 5,000 hospitals). Online directories will be helpful for the many consumers who do not have a regular source of health information or medical care until they get sick.

Hospitals and health plans are employing the Internet to match patients with providers. A growing number of HMOs and health plans offer physician directories, searchable by zip code as well as clinical specialty, such as Anthem Blue Cross and Blue Shield, at anthem-inc .com. One Internet start-up company is organizing a national network of 40,000 physicians to provide house calls for a premium fee. Many of medicine's subspecialists and specialized clinical facilities for such care as oncology, diabetes, plastic surgery, and women's health can be expected to organize virtual chains and market them through the Internet on a national and international basis.

Most Web-browsing healthcare consumers will ultimately choose a local provider, but some patients will use the Internet to find world-class medical organizations with top physicians and research projects. The Internet allows nationally recognized hospitals like Johns Hopkins in Baltimore, Maryland, Houston's MD Anderson, and the Cleveland (Ohio) Clinic to advertise across the nation and internationally.

Health plans and hospitals have been the first to offer provider directories, but other healthcare services are catching up. Consumers seeking information on long-term-care providers can turn to Senior-Place.com, a Portland, Oregon–based firm. We are "building electronic bridges between acute care and long-term care," says Jeff Pentacost, M.D., founder of SeniorPlace (Brock 1998). Offerings from Senior-Place include a patient referral network, listings of providers, and service profiles, with links to web sites of long-term-care providers.

CREATING NEW REVENUE CHANNELS

Dozens of potential applications and electronic commerce opportunities exist for Web-enabled business in the health field, ranging from information display and advertising to online commercial transactions and subscription payments. Many healthcare providers and HMOs have web sites, but few are using the full potential of the Web for electronic commerce. Internet advertising is one of the lowest-cost methods for reaching healthcare consumers. Pharmaceutical companies that are already spending 50 percent of their marketing budgets on direct-to-consumer advertising are expected to migrate their consumer and physician marketing efforts to the Web.

Innovative companies are beginning to demonstrate the commercial potential of the Internet in the health field. The World Wide Web can connect healthcare consumers and providers at a mouse click, expanding healthcare to be a truly global enterprise. In Houston, American Oncology Resources (AOR), a physician practice management company, developed an extranet application, AOR SecureNet, that allows the company's member practices to scan patient information and match patients with clinical trials of advanced cancer treatments (*Businessworld Online* 1999). The first day that one of AOR's practices in Tulsa, Oklahoma had the system installed, it received seven trial matches in different cancers.

Patients and families searching the Web for information about a recent diagnosis or injury bring a higher level of interest to their Internet searches than the average Web surfer. Michael Spector, M.D., of the University Hospital in Cleveland reports, "When you talk to a patient about something major [health problem], they may remember 10 percent. The Internet allows them to ask questions again and get information that was once hard to get without access to a medical library" (Santiago 1998).

Hospital-sponsored foundations are discovering a new way of reaching donors—the Internet. Philanthropy is being reinvented. Healthcare foundations are opening Web pages on their hospitals' web sites, describing programs and soliciting contributions. One Web surfer in the Midwest sent $5,000 to the Cleveland Clinic after a visit to ccf.org, the Clinic's popular web site that attracts 65,000 hits a day and two million hits a month (Santiago 1998). More sophisticated fundraising pitches, like deferred giving, can be introduced on a web site, with follow-up telephone and direct mail response to any Internet consumers expressing interest. Disease-specific fundraising organizations, such as the American Cancer Society and American Foundation for Urologic Disease, are rapidly catching on to the growing use of the Web for health information. Foundations are just a "hot link" away for Internet consumers interested in conditions such as heart disease and breast and prostate cancer.

Online shopping has just begun to focus on healthcare as a broad consumer niche. Health-related products and services likely to be sold widely on the Web include:

- prescription drug refills;
- over-the-counter drugs;
- medical supplies for the chronically ill, for example, diabetics;
- durable medical equipment;
- vitamins and homeopathic medicines; and
- home fitness equipment.

As mentioned earlier in this introduction, pharmaceutical refills have been identified as a high-volume, high-dollar niche that could be just right for the Internet. Mail-order pharmacies may rapidly become obsolete in the face of Internet competitors. Firms like drugstore.com are just getting started, and cvs, the giant national pharmaceutical chain, recently acquired an Internet pharmacy start-up to accelerate its presence in the online retail pharmacy market (Tedeschi 1999). Selling pharmaceuticals requires state licenses, a requirement that has slowed the arrival of online access to drug refills. Once in full swing, online delivery will provide competitive prices, with the deepest discounts available, and the convenience of next-day home delivery. One of the nation's best-known health web sites, drkoop.com, offers pharmaceutical refills and bundles a free "drug checker" software screen for drug compatibility.

INTERNET STRATEGIES FOR MANAGED CARE

Health insurers and HMOs are targeting the Web as a future channel for consumer registration, eligibility verification, and transaction processing. The Internet will be widely used by health plans, hospitals, and large medical groups to provide customer service. Many types of service could be provided online, such as:

- verification of health plan eligibility;
- explanation of health plan benefits;
- search functions for plan-approved providers;
- off-hours access for questions from patients or enrollees;
- requests for referral information, for example, long-term care;
- online registration of new enrollees, for example, a new spouse; and
- notification of changes in status, for example, a new address.

Internet-savvy health insurance customers in the future may shop for a health plan from discount Internet brokers, a Web-enabled market already widely used for online purchase of automobiles, life insurance, and airplane tickets. Consumers enjoy the price savings derived from "disintermediation," that is, cutting out the middleman. Online stock purchases are rising rapidly, accounting for 14 percent of all equity trades in 1998 (*Businessworld Online* 1999).

Web-sold health insurance could become a national business, leapfrogging state and local markets. Internet-empowered consumers have both information and the ability to take their business elsewhere at the click of a mouse. Companies like HealthAxis.com and eHealth-Insurance.com are targeting small employers and the self-insured. For the large employer market, benefits consultants like Towers Perrin and Hewitt are developing electronic insurance options for companies that may switch to defined contribution strategies and allow employees to pick their own health plan option. The biggest health plans and HMOS, which are already licensed in multiple states, could most quickly implement national marketing. Companies like United Healthcare, Aetna U.S. Healthcare, CIGNA, and the Blue Cross–Blue Shield Associations have the multimarket presence and local networks to service customers on a national basis.

At the same time, these big health plans could be vulnerable to new Web-based virtual insurers. These would carry low overhead expenses and would contract at wholesale prices with local provider networks, thus revolutionizing the health insurance market. Medicare HMOS and PPOS could be sold online to a national market of the wired retired, the estimated 40 percent of seniors who now have online access. These national Medicare HMOS could become licensed by the Health Care Financing Administration (HCFA) in every state. [Medicare PPOS are authorized by the Balanced Budget Act (BBA) of 1997 but have not yet been implemented by HCFA.]

Managed care organizations are creating Internet-based help desks to assist consumers in navigating the health system, finding a physician, or checking their health plan's benefits. United Healthcare, based in Minneapolis, Minnesota, offers "Optum Health Forum," a sophisticated web site at which enrollees can search for information, ask about benefits, or check their doctor's status as a participating provider. A web page is vastly cheaper to operate on an hourly basis, notes healthcare consultant Douglas Goldstein, president of Medical Alliances (Baldwin 1998). Other large health insurers like Aetna are investing heavily in providing consumer information and referral through the Web. IntelliHealth, one of the most popular consumer web sites for health information, was initially a joint venture of Aetna with Johns Hopkins. IntelliHealth has now aligned with Harvard to provide the site's medical content.

Predictions for the proliferation of electronic medical records (EMRS) are finally becoming realized. Dozens of companies are offering EMRS. The paper medical chart is not obsolete yet, but the "virtual medical record" is arriving. There are no paperless hospitals in the United States today, but a number of pilot projects are moving forward. At the Woodwinds, a 70-bed hospital in the HealthEast System in St. Paul, Minnesota, executives describe their electronic medical record system as "paper-lite" and hope to become virtually paperless within five years. Medical information will be universally accessible to participating providers in data warehouses with huge electronic storage capacities, which may be operated by payers, providers, or joint plan-provider ventures. In this scenario, patient information can be accessed on a real-time basis for diagnosis and treatment. Health plans and provider-sponsored integrated delivery networks (IDNS) can "mine" their databases to assess and predict risks as well as to measure their medical care against clinical and economic benchmarks. Providers, health plans, and patients can jointly share an EMR housed in a regional data warehouse.

INCREASING EFFICIENCY AND PRODUCTIVITY

The development of intranets and extranets will create dozens of possibilities for expediting business processes and expanding the number of trading partners—physicians, health plans, consumers, and pharmaceutical manufacturers (Businessworld Online 1999). Examples include the following:

- *Clinical trials.* Conducting drug studies and clinical trials is becoming a major industry. Hospital and physician networks can create extranets that directly link patients in trials via the Internet, resulting in a seamless web of telemedicine and clinical research.
- *Clinical protocols.* Hospitals and physicians can share clinical protocols, update algorithms as new research becomes available, track costs and outcomes, communicate with patients, provide reports to health plans and employers, and demonstrate quality improvement.
- *Disease management.* Internet linkages between providers, patients, and disease management programs can improve

outcomes, reduce costs, and prevent early onset of acute symptoms.
- *Clinical variation and cost issues.* The biggest target for Internet-based cost strategies is clinical care. Profiling software can quickly identify cost-effective practitioners using national standards and best-of-breed benchmarks. Health insurers like Indianapolis, Indiana–based Anthem Blue Cross are applying electronic assessment tools in cardiac surgery and only offering contracts to those heart surgery centers that meet Anthem's standards.

Low-cost Internet connectivity is transforming the expensive ($21 billion in 1999) client/server business of traditional legacy information systems (Dornfest 1999). After the frenzied activity surrounding the turn of the century at the year 2000 (Y2K) and the Balanced Budget Act (BBA), many hospitals and medical groups deferred or reduced information systems capital investments by as much as 40 to 60 percent and slashed their information systems (IS) operating costs in 2000 and 2001 below pre-Y2K levels (Hochstadt and Lewis 1999). Capital spending on information technology (IT) will rise again in 2002–2005 as provider organizations spend-up for Health Insurance Portability and Accountability Act (HIPAA)–compliant systems. Deploying Internet technology is being seen as a lower-cost alternative to replacing the legacy health information systems already in place in every hospital and physician office in America. E-health solutions can provide connectivity using the "thin-client" concept, in which vendors own the hardware and may also provide data warehouse storage. In this business model, providers may rent software instead of owning it, paying application service providers (ASPs) for use of the software on a transaction or subscription basis.

BARRIERS TO THE DIGITAL TRANSFORMATION

Although some observers fear the "dot-com-ing" of America, the information age is far from dominant in many parts of the United States. Healthcare providers and health plans seeking to promote their services by Internet linkages may have to wait for some consumers to catch up with the information age. Virtually all American families have a television and a VCR, but many fewer have a personal computer or an Internet connection. One hundred million Americans have regular access to the Web, but they represent barely 40 percent of the total population. Some Web-enabled applications have drawn a quick and positive response, like Napster, a popular music web site with 50 million customers, but many of the dot-coms are struggling to find a viable commercial niche. For e-commerce to reach its full potential, the availability of Internet access must become universal and consumers must be trained in Internet communication skills.

Even if every home had a computer or other Internet access device, some customers still "would prefer to talk to a live person rather than interact with a personal computer," says Doug Whicker, project leader for electronic commerce at Wellmark Blue Cross and Blue Shield in Des Moines, Iowa (Schaich 1999). Market research by Aetna U.S. Healthcare showed that consumers are definitely interested in accessing a web site for service availability information such as physician location, but they are more reluctant to share their medical history or discuss a diagnosis online. To address these concerns, new federal regulations protecting patient privacy in electronic medical records have recently been announced under HIPAA of 1996. Hospitals, doctors, health plans, and pharmacies will have two years to comply with HIPAA regulations, relieving some pressure for wider regulation of Internet consumer privacy by Congress (Simons 1999). HIPAA will be discussed in further detail in chapter 11.

Among the leading barriers that must still be overcome for electronic commerce to be widely employed in healthcare are the following:

- lack of universal Internet access;
- computer illiteracy;
- limited knowledge of how to "surf the Web";
- cost of purchasing computers;
- service costs of online access providers;
- security and confidentiality concerns;
- unwillingness to share personal and medical information;

- unwillingness to put credit card information online;
- compatibility of systems between customer and Web-based organization;
- desire to do business face to face; and
- failure of the organization to array its products or services for online commerce.

The greatest barrier to widespread adoption of e-health strategies may be healthcare's precarious post-BBA finances. Hospitals and health systems experienced their lowest profit margins in five years in 2000, and many are seemingly reluctant to invest heavily in information strategies. A recent survey of academic medical centers by the University Health System Consortium found that 40 percent were losing money and could eventually become clients of the Philadelphia, Pennsylvania–based Hunter Group, a turnaround management company whose recent clients include the University of Pennsylvania and the Stanford University–UC San Francisco Health System (Freudenheim 1999). The Hunter Group typically slashes 15 to 20 percent of capital and operating costs from areas such as information systems.

LOOKING FORWARD: THE DIGITAL TRANSFORMATION OF HEALTHCARE IS HERE

Imagine a world in which consumers make appointments with their physicians online, track their own health history and status in personal electronic medical records, learn about the latest medical research on their conditions, chat with other patients about new drugs, review choices of providers and health plans using Web-based report cards, have access 24 hours a day and seven days a week (24 × 7) to query their doctors and health plans on the Web, and all medical and hospital claims are billed and paid over the Internet. Most of the technology exists to make this scenario a reality today, and it is being rapidly accepted and installed; the Internet revolution in healthcare is here. Utilizing e-health strategies will expand exponentially in the next five years, as America's healthcare executives shift to applying IS and IT to the fundamental business and clinical processes of the healthcare enterprise.

STRATEGIC IMPLICATIONS

The digital transformation of healthcare is arriving at "Internet speed." The arrival of dot-com companies in healthcare seems like only yesterday—and in essence it was. Many e-health enterprises are barely three years old; others did not even survive that long. Apply the following strategies to help ensure Internet-enabled success:

Update Strategic IT Plans. Hospitals, medical groups, health plans, and suppliers must update their strategic information technology plans. Already the new e-health economy is moving into a second generation, escalating past B2C based on mouse clicks and advertising and shifting to industrial-strength B2B strategies, in which revenues are based on transactions or subscriptions.

Initiate Electronic Solutions. Web-based solutions are being applied to both sides of the balance sheet to reduce expenditures and create new revenue sources. Keep an eye on innovators and initiate pilot projects to improve cost and clinical performance.

Gain First-Mover Advantage. For those with capital, digital transformation initiatives clearly reward the market's early movers, who reinvent their market and leave competitors in a cloud of e-dust.

REFERENCES

AMA News. 2001. "More Physicians on the Internet, but Not for Professional Tasks." News Tidbits, February 8, p. 1. [Online news brief.] Southfield, MI: Superior Consultant.

Baldwin, G. 1998. "Pushing the Electronic Envelope: Physicians and Patients Connect Over the Internet." *American Medical News* 41 (28): 19.

Bauer, J. 1999. *Telemedicine and the Reinvention of Healthcare: The Seventh Revolution in Medicine.* New York: McGraw-Hill.

Brock, K. 1998. "Website Offers Long-Term Care Information." *Business Journal–Portland* 15 (27): 6.

Businessworld Online. 1999. "Other Things Equal: How the Internet Is Changing the Economy." [Online article.] *Businessworld Online,* March 2, pp. 1-2.

Business Wire. 2001. "Forrester Research Announces the Birth of the Information Utility." News Briefs, February 28, p. 3. [Online news briefing.] Southfield, MI: Superior Consultant.

Carrns, A. 1999. "Move Over, Drkoop.com: AMA Launches For-Profit Web Venture." *Wall Street Journal,* October 28, p. B4.

Coile, R. C., Jr. 2000. "The Digital Transformation of Health Care." *Physician Executive* January/February: 8–15.

Coile, R. C., Jr., and R. Howe. 1999. "Healthcare Internet and E-Commerce." *Health Trends* 11 (9): 1–12.

Dornfest, S. I. 1999. "The Healthcare Industry in Transition: What It Means to HIT (Health Information Technology) Users and How the Internet Will Help." Presentation materials, Health Internet 2000 Conference, November 1.

Freudenheim, M. 1999. "Bitter Pills for Ailing Hospitals." *New York Times,* October 31, pp. B1, B12–13.

Healtheon. 1999. "Physician Use of the Internet Explodes." *Health Management Technology* 20 (2): 8.

Hochstadt, B., and D. Lewis. 1999. "Bits of Paper to Bytes of Data." White Paper on Healthcare Information and the Internet, pp. 1–66. San Francisco: Thomas Weisel Partners.

Howgill, M. W. 1998. "Health Care Consumerism, the Information Explosion and Branding: Why It's Better to Be the Cowboy than the Cow. *Managed Care Quarterly* 6 (4): 33–43.

Kolata, G. 2001. "Harried Doctors Try to Ease Big Delays and Rushed Visits." *New York Times,* January 4, pp. A1, A16.

Marhula, D. C. 1999. "E-Health: Surf's Up—Time to Catch the Next Wave!" Equity Research Report, pp. 1–40. New York: U.S. Bancorp Piper Jaffray.

Modern Healthcare Daily. 2001. "Losses, Optimism Soar at Medscape." News Tidbits, March 1, pp. 1–2. [Online news briefing.] Southfield, MI: Superior Consultant

Readerman, D. 1999. "E-Health: Can the Internet Cure Malignant Spending?" *Dreaderman's Internet Research Trends (d.i.r.t.),* November 1, pp. 1–8.

Santiago, R. 1998. "Supply and Demand Increase for Internet Health Resources." *Crain's Cleveland Business,* December 7, p. 18.

Schaich, R. L. 1999. "Internet Commerce and Managed Care." *Health Management Technology* 19 (7): 43–47.

Shattuck Hammond Partners. 2000. "E-Health R-Evolution: Tiptoeing ON the Tulips." Research report, pp. 1–27. New York: Shattuck Hammond Partners.

Simons, J. 1999. "New Internet Privacy Laws Appear Less Likely with Release of New Survey." *Wall Street Journal,* May 13, p. B9.

Smith, R. 2001. "E-Business Booster Mary Meeker Becomes E-Lusive." *Wall Street Journal,* March 8, pp. C1, C16.

Tedeschi, B. 1999. "CVS Makes an Internet Move, Acquiring On-Line Drugstore." *New York Times,* May 18, p. C2.

Ukens, C. 1998. "Internet Access Transforming Health Care, Says Koop." *Drug Topics* 142 (22): 80.

Wired Watch. 2000. "Learning More About Medicare." *Dallas Morning News,* May 25, p. 2F.

CHAPTER TWO

Cyber-Health: Transforming Legacy Systems into Enterprise Application Infrastructures

KEY CONCEPTS: *Intranets and extranets • Thin client • Data warehouse • Medical and nursing informatics • Outsourcing • Enterprise application infrastructure*

INTRODUCTION: Healthcare is rapidly converting from analog to digital distribution of information. In the future, all types of information and communication will convert to digital format and merge into one digital stream. Producers of information will have many digital avenues for transmission, and users will be able to customize the information in ways which will transform medical practice and healthcare management (Ruffin 1999). Digital communication will allow the doctor, nurse, or case manager to organize a stream of data (bits) around a specific patient. Somewhere between the high promise of information technology (IT) and the all-too-real performance limitations of today's information systems (IS), every American hospital, medical group, and health system is struggling to upgrade their IS and IT infrastructure to meet the demands of twenty-first-century healthcare. Hospitals and health systems have invested millions in IS and IT, yet many are frustrated with lack of basic functionality. In the past, health organizations beefed up their financial information systems. Now the momentum is swinging to clinical applications and electronic medical records. The five IT applications considered most important in the next two years include clinical information systems, web-based applications, clinical data repositories, computer-based patient records, and point-of-care clinical decision support.

"INFORMATION TECHNOLOGY HAS become mission critical to the cost-efficient delivery of healthcare in the late 1990s; survival is

23

dependent on it. The result is a leap of faith in spending, capital budgets that look like facilities budgets, extreme pressure on the IT organization to deliver, and the acquisition of much new and yet-to-be-proven information technology."

—*Rich Helppie (1998, p. 161)*

The information revolution is sweeping America's hospitals and physician offices, and it will reshape every aspect of its $1.3 trillion healthcare industry. Imagine a medical work station where voice, broadcast-quality video, three-dimensional (3-D) graphics, color photographs and images, and even animation are all available at the click of a mouse in online electronic medical records. In fact, the model already exists at the University of Pittsburgh, built with a $2.5 million grant from the National Library of Medicine (Monahan 1997). Patient care will never be the same.

THE DIFFERENCE IS DIGITAL

Society is rapidly converting from analog to digital distribution of information. In the future, all types of information and communication will convert to digital format and merge into one digital stream. Producers of information will have many digital avenues for transmission, and users can customize the information in ways that will transform medical practice and healthcare management, predicts Marshall Ruffin in *Digital Doctors* (1999). Digital communication will allow the doctor, nurse, or case manager to organize a stream of data (bits) around a specific patient. A doctor will have an automated search program that provides a daily synopsis of the latest medical literature in his or her field from the National Library of Medicine. A physician or care worker will make rounds with a preformatted set of information displayed on a handheld computer for each patient and updated with wireless communication. In this "post-information" age, data are mass customized for each user.

Yet these futuristic developments for healthcare is and it are still overcoming buyer skepticism. Somewhere between the high promise of information technology and the all-too-real performance limitations of today's information systems, every American hospital, medical group, and health system is struggling to upgrade its is and it infrastructure to meet the demands of twenty-first-century healthcare. Hospitals and health systems have invested millions in is and it, yet many are frustrated with lack of basic functionality, such as local area networks (LANS) to provide universal patient registration and information architecture for all users. In the past, health organizations beefed up their financial information systems. Now the momentum is swinging to clinical applications and electronic medical records. According to the latest Leadership Survey by the Health Information Management Systems Society of Chicago, the five it applications considered most important in the next two years are (HIMSS 2001):

1. clinical information systems;
2. Web-based applications;
3. a clinical data repository;
4. computer-based patient records; and
5. point-of-care clinical decision support.

THE 100 MOST-WIRED HOSPITALS

A gap is emerging and growing between the early adopters of technology and the rest of the health industry. The American Hospital Association (AHA) designates the "100 Most-Wired" institutions as those that have the information infrastructure and Internet interfaces to manage many functions electronically and at a lower cost (Solovy 2000). In a national survey of hospitals and health systems, the most-wired facilities are much more deeply involved with e-commerce than their less-wired counterparts. One in four of the most-wired hospitals use the Internet for more than 80 percent of supply-chain transactions, compared with only one in nine less-wired institutions. Managed care business transactions are being migrated to the Web; more than 20 percent of the most-wired hospitals routinely accomplish precertifications and referral authorizations electronically.

The most-wired hospitals have established Internet linkages with their patients and medical staff. One in ten of the most-wired hospitals is already scheduling appointments online, and two in three are making physician referrals on the Web. Almost 80 percent of the most wired are hot linked to patient support groups, and 58 percent of them offer online access to patient data to their medical staff. Doctors in these hospitals also get online decision support, laboratory order entry and results, and radiology consultations over the Web or through hospital-sponsored intranets.

The good news for the less-wired institutions is that they can move rapidly to become electronically connected and enabled. In Gallup, New Mexico, the Rehoboth McKinley Christian Hospital "was so far behind we were out of sight," claims CIO Dwayne Jordan. However, the hospital was able to make the most-wired list after two years of investment, "a quantum leap in technology, going from the back of the pack to the front" (Solovy 2000, p. 32).

INFORMATION SYSTEMS ARE A STRATEGIC IMPERATIVE

Most healthcare chief executives are selling their boards on the strategic value of information systems investments (see Figure 2.1). Despite the lack of a short-term payoff, most hospitals and health systems believe they cannot resist this strategic imperative, according to the Leadership Survey of 1,200 healthcare IS and IT professionals conducted by HIMSS (Cochrane 1998). One of the rationales for multihospital integrated systems has been standardizing information systems; however, integrating these systems after mergers or acquisitions often results in increased capital spending. Consolidating IS or IT operations may result in savings, but obtaining cost cuts from combining information systems staff and support functions may take three to five years to achieve. University of California, Berkeley–based health services researcher Stephen Shortell has studied integrated delivery systems

Figure 2.1: Justifying Information Systems Expenditures

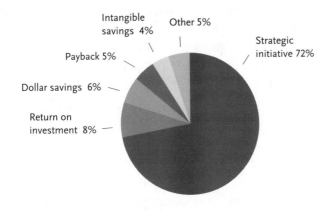

Source: Adapted from Morrisey (1998a, p. 71).

for ten years; his conclusion is not encouraging: "In spite of millions, if not billions, of dollars spent on information systems, none of the information systems of these healthcare systems is sufficiently developed to where it is a true asset for physician and clinical integration" (Shortell et al. 2000, p. 39). On an integration scale of 1 to 5, information technology integration ranked only a 2.7.

IS- AND IT-INVESTMENT IS THE BRIDGE TO THE TWENTY-FIRST CENTURY

Information technology performance in healthcare organizations is not yet what it needs to be. When 300-bed hospitals prepare a strategic IT plan and find the price tag will be $15 to $20 million, the CEO and board may reasonably question whether they will get $15 to $20 million of value for this investment. The answer is, there is no good alternative to making this (or an even higher) capital investment.

In hospital after hospital, providers are struggling to upgrade their outdated legacy information systems. Other providers have decided to replace their core systems and are considering other capital investments in new is and it, which may cost the hospital $25 to $40 million or more in the next five years. But will these substantial is and it investments repay their hospitals or medical groups with improved cost management or revenue capture? Today, allocating capital spending on information technology is still a leap of faith for many healthcare executives. Market observer John Morrisey believes ceos are believers in the promise of information systems; they have faith the hefty spending will pay off, but many are waiting for tangible results before committing their financial resources (Morrisey 1998a, p. 70).

Capital investments for information systems are too strategic—and too expensive—to be made by technical staff and chief information officers. Across the nation, $11.6 billion was spent in 1996 on health information systems, with 61 percent in acute care settings. Total healthcare is and it expenditures may have risen to $18 billion during 2000, according to recent industry estimates (Dorenfest 1997). Multimillion dollar expenditures for is and it have climbed to the top of capital budgets for America's 5,300 community hospitals and 350 integrated health systems. A 1998 survey on is trends found approximately 75 percent of final is and it decisions are made by ceos and boards (Morrisey 1998a).

Across the nation, spending on health information systems is rising. About 40 percent of hospitals and health systems in *Modern Healthcare*'s annual survey are spending less than 2 percent of budget on information systems (Morrisey 1998a). Many hospitals and health systems are merely attempting to catch up to major is and it upgrades. More than 10 percent of provider organizations are now targeting 5 percent of their operating budgets for is operations and capital investments. In a similar survey published in February 1998 by himss, one-third of providers plan to boost is and it expenditures by more than 20 percent in 2001 (himss 1998).

The average hospital spends 2.55 percent of its budget on is and it, according to the *Modern Healthcare* survey. Spending for is and it is

Figure 2.2: IS Priorities in the Next Two Years

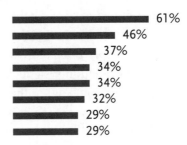

Upgrade security/HIPAA compliance	61%
Deploy Internet technology	46%
Improve IS cost-effectiveness	37%
Upgrade network infrastructure	34%
Upgrade inpatient clinical systems	34%
Implement electronic data interchange	32%
Implement CPR system	29%
Upgrade financial systems	29%

Source: HIMSS (2001, p. 14).

still increasing; 94 percent of hospitals and health systems plan to increase information systems expenditures in 2002 (Morrisey 1998a, p. 76). Costs for upgrading and operating healthcare IS and IT systems are rising 15 percent each year, an increase that does not include low-level departmental expenditures for desktop computers, notebook computers, software, and LANs (Helppie 1998).

ENTERPRISE MANAGEMENT

Enterprisewide information systems are critical to embracing the management of large regional delivery networks by creating competitive advantage and improving productivity. Managing virtual organizations requires expanding from LANs to WANs—wide-area networks—that link providers across a market region or a nation (Joch 1998). Health system managers envision a "dashboard" of management indicators that will provide real-time information on issues such as compliance monitoring or staff overtime.

Improving every health organization's finances is still a major goal of IS and IT, especially as hospital net income fell below 2 percent in 1999. Managed care contract administration is a strategic essential that has demonstrated short-term benefits from IS investments (see Figure 2.2). Payer-based cost data are essential for negotiating managed care contracts, especially in arrangements involving risk and capitation. Hospitals also hope to gain improved productivity and cost reductions through integration of databases. Increasing accuracy of charge capture in patient accounting, boosting cash flow, and improving collections are important incentives for automating cost data. Upgrading financial information systems is still an important priority, but HIPAA compliance, deploying for the Internet, and clinical management applications are now getting management's top attention.

Hospitals and health systems are taking advantage of expert systems that can automate management tasks such as variable staffing on a daily or even hourly basis. Environmental services and energy management are another area for automated systems management. In the future, expect to see health systems use experts for management functions such as continuous performance assessment of clinical product lines or nursing units, customer service monitoring and improvement, and online staff continuing education and training.

In the pharmacy, automated decentralized pharmacy dispensing systems (ADPDSS) are being installed in growing numbers (ECRI 1997). The automated systems include one or several computer-controlled dispensing cabinets interfaced with a central computer in the pharmacy. For an investment of less than $200,000, a hospital may put automated dispensing cabinets on four units, reducing labor and transportation costs and improving control over pharmacy costs and narcotics use.

ELECTRONIC LINKAGES

Electronic linkages are moving buyers, sellers, and competitors into new relationships. The future potential of digital, Internet-enabled commerce is just now being tapped. Today's global revenues of $26 billion for electronic commerce are predicted to soar to $1 trillion by the year 2005, according to economists for the Organization of Economic Cooperation and Development (OCED) in London (Strassel 1998). In the past three years, Internet commerce has revolutionized niche markets and created new marketing, sales, and distribution channels for companies like Amazon.com, which became America's fifth largest bookseller in five years. OCED analysts note that 70 percent of all retail sales are typically generated by 30 percent of the customers. On the Internet, Web-based shoppers tend to be wealthy, upwardly mobile professionals who are short on time and likely to buy via the Internet for convenience.

Thus, the Internet is reinventing managed care relationships. Providers are increasingly reliant on electronic claims submission: some 60 percent of all provider claims are now submitted electronically (Anderson 1998). Hospitals are even more dependent on electronic claims, with 83 percent of all claims sent via electronic data interchange (EDI). Some 86 percent of pharmacy claims are now submitted electronically. However, physician offices lag behind the trend: only 36 percent of physician office charges were sent electronically to payers.

Hospitals are contributing to this trend by creating electronic linkages between and among their medical staffs. After the costly failures of acquiring physicians in the 1990s, many hospitals are focusing on two new priorities: building clinical communication into healthcare delivery systems and using the Web as a lower-cost strategy for rebuilding the hospital-physician relationship. Links to physicians are now leading the list of strategies for developing integrated delivery systems, according to *Modern Healthcare*'s annual survey of healthcare executives (Kirchheimer 2001). In Houston, Texas, the 12-hospital Memorial Hermann Health System has developed a physician-centered intranet, which is hosted by an application service provider called Healthvision. Based in Dallas, Healthvision hosts Hermann Memorial and other hospitals' intranets from a data center in New Jersey.

Transactions are just one application of telecommunications and computer databases. In the future, expect significant development in the following areas:

- IDN-shared information systems;
- regional data warehouses;
- electronic commerce;
- electronic claims and payment;
- automated consumer verification;
- 60-second treatment authorization;

- continuous inventory or just-in-time supply; and
- report card–type information, for example, Health Plan Employer Data and Information Set (HEDIS) data.

EMERGING TECHNOLOGIES

At the intersection of medical science and computer technology, a new set of integrated decision-support systems are emerging that could revolutionize diagnosis and treatment. One example is the University of Pittsburgh's "Image Engine" (Monahan 1997). Under development since 1994, the university's new technologies bring together complex data from patient records, taking full advantage of today's vastly more powerful computer systems. Sophisticated graphics software is being used to present dynamic images in 3-D and full animation. Patient information is compiled from enterprise record systems or from public Internet data available through services such as Medline. Researchers at Pitt have also developed their own Internet browser, called Web-Report, for accessing multimedia clinical information, which is now being installed at the university's Cancer Institute.

Many of the implements for tomorrow's information technology, such as e-mail, the Internet, networks of personal computers, and computer-based clinical decision-support systems, have been available for years. Still, many hospitals and health systems are only beginning to link all services and settings into an integrated information environment. Physician offices are even further behind in joining the information age. Data from the 1998 HIMSS study, shown in Figure 2.3, identify emerging technologies that CIOs expect to be implemented in their organizations in the immediate future (HIMSS 1998; Serb 1998).

A major barrier to information integration—hardware and software incompatibility—is now being overcome. The rapidly spreading use of "object-orientation" software like Java offers a way for hospitals and health systems with old-fashioned legacy information systems to integrate years-old software with modern hardware. Java applications can run on any computer platform, from Microsoft Windows to Unix to Macintosh. Sun Microsystems, Java's developer, estimates that 450

Figure 2.3: "Infoagenda" for IS and IT in the Future—Applications to Be Implemented in the Next 12 Months

Voice recognition	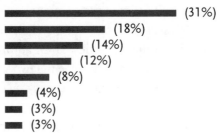 (31%)
Wireless information appliances	(18%)
Web-enabled applications	(14%)
Handheld PDAs for workgroups	(12%)
Telecom links to patients homes	(8%)
Component-based architecture	(4%)
Enterprisewide patient records	(3%)
Object-oriented technology	(3%)

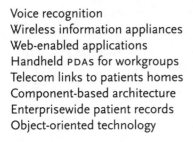

Source: Adapted from HIMSS (1998).

independent software vendors are developing applications with Java, exemplifying its "write once, run anywhere" slogan (Monahan 1997). Other areas that promise to revolutionize the healthcare industry include voice recognition, artificial intelligence, and even a national healthcare "extranet," which could create a national clinical database available to every healthcare provider (Heimoff 1998).

TEN TRENDS FOR HEALTHCARE INFORMATION SYSTEMS

Trend 1—HIPAA

After months of delay and wrangling, new federal regulations to ensure the privacy of electronic medical records are now moving forward. HIPAA, passed in 1996, was intended to standardize electronic commerce in healthcare, but federal regulators acting barely a month before the end of the Clinton administration carried the rules much further. The final regulations require that most providers get patients' signed consent for routine use and disclosure of health records, a tighter standard than the draft regulations, which would have allowed routine disclosures without advance consent. The new rules were also expanded to cover paper as well as electronic medical records, in anticipation that paper records will eventually be digitized.

Providers reacted strongly. The proposed regulations attracted more than 52,000 comments, many from hospitals and physicians complaining about the expense and disruption that full HIPAA compliance would require. The new Bush administration may revise the regulations, adding more time to the two-year implementation deadline and easing some of the more costly and complex HIPAA rules proposed by Clinton-era regulators.

Consultants may benefit from a mini-boom in information services assistance to meet HIPAA requirements. In a study for AHA, a price tag of $20 to $25 billion was projected for upgrading and consulting expenditures to meet HIPAA standards. Some 61 percent of the nation's health information managers rate HIPAA their highest priority in 2001, according to the latest Leadership Survey by HIMSS (2001). Despite plenty of warnings that the task is huge and time lines short, market observers believe that getting healthcare executives to make HIPAA their top priority could be an uphill battle (Morrisey 2001a). Hospitals are still occupied with Web-enabling their organizations, and implementing clinical information systems and electronic medical records are very important to their medical staff.

Trend 2—Upgrading Legacy Systems

During the last 10 to 15 years, hospitals and integrated delivery systems have spent an estimated $100 billion on legacy information systems, according to Wall Street analysts at U.S. Bancorp Piper Jaffray (Hochstadt and Lewis 1999). Continued demands for IT capital have caused healthcare executives to complain, "It's almost an endless hole" (Morrisey 1998b). After spending millions of dollars to upgrade systems to meet Y2K, hospitals are now facing the prospect of spending millions more to become HIPAA compliant. But most CEOs believe they must beef up their information systems or fall behind competitors and the market in building an information architecture sufficiently robust to manage future demands.

Figure 2.4: Hospitals Use Multiple Software and Hardware

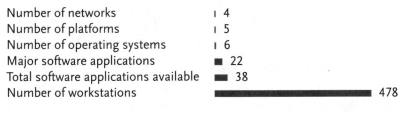

Number of networks	ı 4
Number of platforms	ı 5
Number of operating systems	ı 6
Major software applications	■ 22
Total software applications available	▬ 38
Number of workstations	▬▬▬▬▬▬▬▬▬▬▬▬ 478

Source: Adapted from Anderson (1997).

Wall Street analyst Bruce Hochstadt, M.D., predicts that hospitals will invest in "enterprise application infrastructure," which will liberate legacy systems and increase performance using the following (Hochstadt 2001, p. 11):

- improved performance of critical hardware and software functionality;
- business process automation;
- Internet-based communications (HIPAA secure);
- applications integration across the extended enterprise; and
- real-time data analysis to reengineer business and clinical processes.

Hospitals of all sizes are incorporating electronic medical records, remote order entry, and universal registration systems. But few institutions or systems are using a standardized single vendor or integrated solution. In a recent study of 600 hospital information systems departments by Health Data Management in San Ramon, California, market researchers found that hospitals are purchasing or upgrading software packages and hardware platforms from multiple vendors. The average hospital is using dozens of software applications daily (see Figure 2.4).

Operating a hospital is department is expensive, even in small hospitals. The average (median) annual operating expense for a hospital is department is $741,643, according to the Health Data Management national survey, and ranged from $273,909 to $1,914,568 (Anderson 1997). Information systems staff work an average of 1.61 hours per discharge, at a cost of $81.47 for every inpatient.

Trend 3—Clinical Information Systems

Better clinical information—not cost information—may be the ultimate bottom line for healthcare is and it initiatives. The long-term value of mega-investments in is and it may be better clinical care management. Clinical decision making, linking costs of care to outcomes, and improving patient care capabilities are important priorities for health systems development, and physician acceptance is the critical watershed factor. As physicians increasingly use automated health information systems and electronic medical records, they will find more value to the clinical process. The trend could lead to the creation of a new position, "chief medical information officer" (cmio), for physicians with a strong background in medical informatics who would have charge of the clinical information system. In the next five years, the role of the hospital's or health system's chief medical officer (cmo) will be increasingly important in selecting and spending for clinical information systems.

In twenty-first-century healthcare, megamemory clinical work stations may be supplemented—or replaced—by thin-client server technology that taps the power of Web-based applications with network computers holding only 8 mb of core memory and costing only $400 to $750. Doctors and nurses will be able to conduct rounds and enter and receive patient data with pocket computers that weigh less than one pound and are tuned to limited-use telecommunications channels. High-speed networks using asymmetric digital subscriber loop (adsl) modem technology may blast information at rates of 1.5 to 8 mb per second over existing telephone lines, much faster than a current isdn line at 128 kilobytes per second. Accessing an x-ray or computerized axial tomography (ct) scan could take a doctor only seconds, not minutes or hours as is the case now.

Trend 4—Web-Based Applications

The World Wide Web is transforming healthcare. Hospitals and health systems are creating intranets of Web communications within their organizations, as well as extranets that create direct linkages with outside organizations, such as physician offices, suppliers, or payers (Nussbaum 1997). E-mail has rapidly become universal in hospitals and health systems. No longer just a communications tool, Internet-based networks are now the repository for clinical and financial data, policies and procedures, and many types of electronic transactions such as ordering and billing.

Trend 5—Electronic Medical Records

Privacy and security concerns as well as cost and complexity are slowing the diffusion of electronic medical records. Only 2 percent of CIOs and CEOs completing the annual HIMSS survey in February 1998 have a fully electronic medical records system in place. Improvements in clinical and financial information systems have raised hopes that soon paperless health systems may be a reality. Mayo's new hospital in Scottsdale, Arizona, which opened in Fall 1998, may become the nation's first fully paperless hospital after making a $100 million IT investment and training 3,500 health workers and physicians.

The future of electronic medical records is picking up momentum, but a number of issues need to be addressed, including:

- patient confidentiality;
- provider privacy and security;
- universal patient registration;
- systemwide information access;
- remote order entry;
- personal electronic medical records;
- multisite clinical research studies;
- longitudinal health assessment; and
- smart cards or implanted devices.

Trend 6—Point-of-Care Clinical Decision-Support Systems

Expert systems and clinical databases are producing powerful medical management tools. Automation of clinical pathways and protocols is accelerating. Information industry observer Steve Heimoff believes, "Computerization is a strategic decision. In order to provide quality care in the future, you have to know what's going on with your patient" (Heimoff 1998, p. 14). As the new millennium progresses, doctors and nurses will be using automated medical decision-support systems to diagnose illness and manage patient care.

This is not a prediction for "electronic medical cookbooks." Medical informatics consultants note that clinicians are encouraged to override the medical knowledge system's suggestions whenever appropriate (Lando 1998). Computerized clinical decision-support systems will help doctors trying to cope with "several feet of protocols" to analyze the most relevant patient data, restoring responsibility for care back to the clinician and relieving HMOs from having to make decisions about care (Solberg 1998, p. 36).

Clinical managers will have a dashboard of clinical quality indicators that signal when care processes are not performed to benchmark standards. The goal is to reduce costly variation in medical treatment and improve clinical outcomes. Clinical care and cost management improve when clinicians have access to real-time patient information. In a recent study by Utah-based InterMountain Healthcare, patients at Salt Lake City's LDS Hospital who were treated by physicians using bedside computers got well quicker, suffered fewer complications, and were discharged sooner (Cochrane 1998, p. 18).

Enhanced clinical information systems can improve quality assurance and provide the data record for regulatory compliance activities. Medical utilization management and optimized care efficiency will also be facilitated and improved. For example, pharmacy management can identify drug incompatibility problems for patients, as well as identify opportunities for therapeutic interchange of generic or lower-cost drugs over brand-name prescriptions.

Many hospitals and at-risk provider organizations are installing electronic "demand management" programs. Using regional call centers and toll-free telephone access, patients can be triaged and channeled to the appropriate provider setting and service or simply be given health information that they can use to manage their own health conditions at home (Lando 1998). Risk management of chronically ill patients is an especially promising large-scale application. Scanning databases of health histories and past utilization, at-risk providers and health plans can identify the 12 to 15 percent of seniors and 6 to 8 percent of under-65 adults who are likely to experience costly healthcare needs.

Trend 7—Telemedicine

Telemedicine is gaining acceptance as cost-effective medical technology. Early pilot projects focused on rural health and emergency medicine and demonstrated the feasibility of the technology, but at per-patient costs of $500 to $1,000 per encounter. Now telemedicine applications are shifting into mainstream medicine with off-site clinical consultation and regional medical referral networks. Telemedicine is not just a rural health strategy. In urban Los Angeles, the Charles R. Drew University of Medicine has just opened its third telemedicine clinic, a pediatric clinic in South Central Los Angeles (Tieman 2001). Two ophthalmology clinics are already in operation in public housing projects in East Los Angeles and Long Beach. The network of five telemedicine clinics has been started with foundation funding and a grant from the Los Angeles County Development Commission. A billing mechanism is being developed that should help bring in patient care revenues by 2002.

Medical advice is now available on the Internet but is not currently compensated through insurance. This lack of payment from insurers is a significant hurdle still to be overcome: Medicare, for example, requires face-to-face sessions between physicians and patients. Interactive videoconferences do not qualify for payment. Cross-border licensing issues, security, and legal liability concerns are also holding back the development of online medical practice at this time. Providers and payers can expect new federal legislation to address telemedicine issues within the next two to three years.

Teleradiology is one of the fastest-growing medical applications of telecommunications. Despite legal liability and physician licensure issues, teleradiology is becoming widely used for subspecialty consultations and off-site reading of images by on-call radiologists. The costs of expanding teleradiology are not inexpensive. Hardware costs for a single image capture and receiving station can range from $15,000 to $80,000, not including hardware and software maintenance and system operating costs. Beyond teleradiology, future telemedicine applications may include (ECRI 1997):

- telementoring of surgeons;
- advanced healthcare delivery to underdeveloped regions;
- home monitoring of critically ill patients; and
- remote control of robotic-assisted surgery.

Telemedicine networks have already become established as low-cost, accessible channels for continuing education. Distance is no barrier to sharing education programs or conducting grand rounds as part of global clinical education conferences. The Internet can also be used for prevention and health promotion. In addition, drug interaction monitoring systems are widely used by HMOs, health insurers, and pharmacy benefit managed care organizations (PBMCOs).

Trend 8—Cyber-Marketing

Online communications and powerful databases are being linked for strategic marketing and competitive advantage. Marketers are hooking together new retail-oriented consumer tactics by employing web sites, the Internet, "push" technology, and computerized databases. Healthcare organizations have been slow to adopt the Internet beyond creating web sites that are little more than "electronic brochures." Jeff Goldsmith, president of HealthFutures in Charlottesville, Virginia, observes that hospitals are still operating in the "old economy," whereas the Internet and information technology are transforming the "new economy" (Goldsmith 2001). The best use of the Internet is not to market the hospital but to make using the hospital easier and more transparent to consumers.

Jeff Goldsmith suggests that a personal health record (PHR) may be a key marketing strategy for the future (Goldsmith 2001), and the Internet makes this possible. Individuals may create and maintain their own PHRs in the future, and hospitals, physicians, and health plans will supply patients with a personal health web site. Denver-based WebFamilies has launched an early effort, recently signing up 50 Tenet and HCA hospitals for an Internet-based service that provides maternity patients with the ability to create password-protected web sites chronicling their children's births (Flory 2001). Patients may send digital photographs of their newborns and text messages directly to the Web, where family members can remotely access them.

Other features of a PHR include the following:

- Data from patient care, diagnostic tests, and treatment outcomes can be electronically forwarded to the patients' PHRs.
- Internet-linked health monitoring equipment can allow home-bound patients to maintain a continuous record of their health status and transmit the information to providers, case managers, or disease management organizations.
- Internet connections will allow patients to interact with providers and health plans through their personal health web sites.
- Patients can schedule visits to physicians, supply medical and financial data, and receive test results, self-health information, and the latest findings from the medical literature. This electronic record can also be backed up on a medical smart card.

Future trends in healthcare cyber-commerce include:

- database marketing;
- psychogeodemographics;
- clinical research protocols and test panels;
- market research and product development;
- physician directories and provider referrals;

- direct-to-consumer marketing;
- online advertising; and
- e-commerce—selling, for example, durable medical equipment.

Trend 9—Outsourcing

Rising capital expenditures and staff shortages are accelerating IT and IS outsourcing. The outsourcing trend for IT and IS climbed 11.5 in 1998, according to *Modern Healthcare*'s annual contracting survey (Ngeo 1998). In addition, departmental outsourcing contracts jumped 45 percent in a variety of administrative and clinical areas.

Cost reduction is usually the primary goal. Outsourcing IS and IT at Cedars-Sinai in Los Angeles, for example, saved 20 percent of operating costs and slashed capital costs by $1.5 billion (Luevanos 1997). Providers are definitely interested in reducing costs, but the main attraction of the outsourcing model is selling based on its potential to improve quality and to consolidate nonclinical services across a healthcare system. In Evanston, Illinois, the three-hospital Evanston Northwestern Healthcare system has a combined IT and telecommunications budget of $16 million, much of which is now managed under a new outsourcing arrangement with McKesson/HBOC (Morrisey 2001b). The outsourcing agreement helped increase income from operations in 2000, which jumped 60 percent to $23 million on net operating income of $711 million. The Evanston hospital has placed among the top 100 hospitals in the United States for the past seven years.

Hospitals and health systems have four options for outsourcing their IS and IT departments, including the following:

1. *Data center and technology outsourcing.* The outsourcing vendor staffs and operates the data center or moves the functions to a consolidated off-site data center, leaving only support staff on-site.
2. *Applications outsourcing.* The vendor assumes responsibility for supporting, maintaining, and improving the current applications systems and for implementing new applications.

3. *Help desk.* The outside firm takes responsibility for providing technical assistance and support services on a 24-hour by seven-day (24 × 7) basis for maintaining the hospital's or system's computer network or specific applications.
4. *Total outsourcing.* The vendor takes full responsibility for all is and IT functions, including data center, applications, operations, capital budget, staffing, hardware and software upgrades, trouble-shooting, and system development (e.g., intranets and extranets).

The concept of "capitated consulting" by outsourcing is and IT shifts risk to vendors to control increases in staff, equipment, and consulting costs (Helppie 1998). Under at-risk outsourcing arrangements, hospitals can control the often unpredictable costs of managing and upgrading IT systems. Outsourcing also addresses two of the highest concerns identified by a recent HIMSS Leadership Survey of healthcare executives, including recruiting and retention of quality employees and integrating systems from multiple vendors (Serb 1998). Outsourcing offers career upward mobility and CIO recruitment and retention and puts the burden on the outsourcing vendor to solve the ongoing problem of staffing shortages of technicians. Vendors must implement technology updates and hardware and software installation without disrupting the operations of the organization.

Physician linkages are another focus of contracting electronic strategies to outside vendors. Outsourcing can provide a solution to building intranets linking physicians. Houston-based Memorial Hermann Health System has outsourced its physician intranet, called Physicianlink, to Healthvision, a Dallas-based healthcare Internet company (Kirchheimer 2001). The goal is to provide a set of Internet applications to doctors that facilitate the management of patients. The Physicianlink system can be customized so physicians can quickly access sites of particular interest or view information organized to the needs of their specialty. Some 1,000 physicians participate in Memorial Hermann's intranet, which serves as a key strategy for building physician loyalty, now that Memorial Hermann has spun off its employed physician network.

HIPAA will also drive more outsourcing in the health field. As the two-year time line for the HIPAA compliance deadline begins in 2001, some hospitals and health systems are bringing in outsourcing vendors to provide HIPAA solutions. Delegating HIPAA compliance to the outsourcing vendor means the company can move quickly to assess the HIPAA status of mission-critical systems without disrupting business operations while organizing long-term solutions to HIPAA process, policy, and training issues.

Trend 10—Smart Cards

More than nine million "smart cards" are in use across the nation, but experts still call this device a "technology solution looking for a problem" (Dugas 1998, p. B1). Smart cards could be used by health insurers and HMOs to store plan eligibility information and health data, but few health plans have implemented them on a large scale. However, the computer chip–based cards are finding wider uses and may replace cash some day. A widely watched experiment on New York's West Side, however, found relatively few users for a smart card marketed jointly by Chase Manhattan Bank and Citibank. Consumers were encouraged to transfer funds from their bank accounts onto smart cards and use the cards for small cash purchases with local merchants. But many New Yorkers said it was simpler to just use cash.

Commercial applications of smart cards are growing, however. In healthcare, users include health plans, hospitals, and health systems, but medical smart cards are still not in widespread circulation. On college campuses, smart cards are becoming more widely accepted, as schools combine an identification card and cash card together. Smart cards are also used to prepay long-distance telephone charges. Citibank hopes to broaden acceptance of its cash smart cards by selling consumers a "personal ATM" for only $8.95, which could be used in conjunction with a personal computer to download and transfer cash from bank accounts to cash cards.

LOOKING FORWARD: OVERCOMING E-SKEPTICISM

Although skeptics worry about drowning in too much information or spending millions of dollars on systems that do not work, mounting evidence shows that IS and IT investments are paying off in improved productivity and patient outcomes. In Walnut Creek, California, nurses at the John Muir Medical Center save steps and labor costs by routinely using portable computers for data entry and patient management (Heimoff 1998). Some 350 wireless personal computers, called "slates," are placed throughout the hospital. Nurses and physicians use a point-and-click stylus to record data in templates of pre-designed notes in a system designed by Atlanta-based HBOC, a national healthcare information technology firm. Data are electronically beamed to overhead sensors, which pass them along the hospital's mainframe computer. Caregivers can pull up a week's worth of data in graphic form, a capability which allows observers to spot trends and patterns.

Wireless technology will transform communications and electronic data interchange, from room-size "personal area networks" to globe-spanning telecommunications, predicts Matt Hite of Woodstream Consulting in Nicholasville, Kentucky (Hite 2001). At the short-range end of the spectrum, Bluetooth is a wireless network designed to operate within 10 to 25 feet and at speeds of up to 10 Mbps. Communication can be hands free with an earbud microphone to a cell phone or personal digital assistant (PDA). This solution will link PDA-sized hand-held electronic medical records on a nursing unit, surgical suite, or physician office. Wireless LANs expand the range of connectivity to typically a building or a campus. WANs provide wireless intercommunications among devices and services located anywhere, connecting hospitals and other care sites into integrated health systems. A new generation of cellular telephones will work in hospitals just like conventional wired phones. Based on a new set of standards called third generation (3G), specially built wireless telephones will act just like wired phones, with multiple lines, call forwarding, and voice mail features.

This kind of progress will not occur overnight. Significant capital investments, staff training, and process improvement will be needed to obtain real payoffs from today's IS and IT initiatives. Tomorrow's healthcare information systems will not only provide data faster and cheaper; automated healthcare IS and IT will provide decision support to improve the accuracy of physician diagnosis and the outcomes of nursing care management. Twenty-first-century medicine can cope with the knowledge explosion in only one way: investment in IS and IT now.

STRATEGIC IMPLICATIONS

The health field is moving toward a digital transformation, but not yet at Internet speed. Healthcare providers are typically slow to adopt new technology and are often more concerned about avoiding risk than being first movers.

Align E-Strategies with Overall Strategies. Think of information technology and the Internet as the "Intel inside" of every market and operations strategy. Like Intel's chips, which power computers, e-strategies can facilitate the achievement of every hospital strategic goal.

CEOs and COOs Must "Own" Their Hospital's IT Strategy. Futurist Jeff Goldsmith argues that CEOS must make implementing a customer-friendly network computing environment their number-one or number-two priority. COOs must embrace network computing applications as a vehicle for improving efficiency and customer service, and CEOS and COOS must shed their aversion to computing and become IT-literate change-management advocates.

Invest in an IT-Driven Future. Delivering healthcare in the future will be an electronically enabled process, from the critical care unit to the "hospital in the home." Every aspect of medicine and health will be touched by information technology and connected by the Internet. Healthcare organizations need a long-term vision for building an information infrastructure that will support the highest quality care coordinated across multiple settings. This requires a capital budget and a sustained investment during the next ten years, in partnership with IT suppliers and consultants who can provide the state-of-the-art technology and best practices in the employment of information systems.

References

Anderson, H. J. 1997. "Comparing Hospital I.S. Departments." *Health Data Management* February: 134.

Anderson, H. 1998. "Trends in Health Care Information Technology." *Health Data Directory*, 1997–1998 edition, pp. 7–20.

Cochrane, J. 1998. "1998 Information Systems Priorities." *Integrated Healthcare Report* 5 (1): 17–19,

Dorenfest, S. I. 1997. "A Look Behind the Rapid Growth in Healthcare IS." *Healthcare Informatics* June: 29–30.

Dugas, C. 1998. "Smart Cards Dumb Idea? Value of Using Card Over Cash Lost on Consumers." *USA Today*, September 22, pp. B1, B2.

ECRI. 1997. "Health Technology Forecast." *Healthcare Information Systems* July: 61–63.

Flory, J. 2001. "Web Scan: Tenet and HCA Sign Up Hospitals for WebFamilies." *Internet Healthcare Strategies* 3 (1): 12.

Goldsmith, J. C. 2001. "How Hospitals Should Be Using the Internet." *Healthcare Market Strategist* 2 (1): 1, 15–18.

Healthcare Information Management Systems Society (HIMSS). 1998. "Ninth Annual HIMSS Leadership Survey." *Healthcare Informatics* May: 55–74.

———. 2001. "12th Annual HIMSS Leadership Survey." Preliminary results, pp. 1–28. Chicago: HIMSS.

Heimoff, S. 1998. "The Forces that Impact Healthcare—Technology." *Healthcare Forum Journal* 40 (1): 14–19.

Helppie, R. D. 1998. "Bring in the Ringer: Should Your Organization Consider Outsourcing?" *Healthcare Informatics* February: 161–68.

Hite, M. 2001. "Wireless Voice Systems: Beyond the Cell Phone." *Spectrum* 1 (2): 1–2.

Hochstadt, B. 2001. "E-Commerce Truths and Consequences for Hospital and Health Systems Boards." Presentation materials, February 6, pp. 1–12. La Jolla, CA: The Governance Institute.

Hochstadt, B., and D. Lewis. 1999. "Bits of Paper to Bytes of Data." White Paper on Healthcare Information and Internet, October 27, pp. 1–66. San Francisco: Thomas Weisel Partners.

Joch, A. 1998. "Wiping the Slate Clean: Why Network Outsourcing Is In." *Healthcare Informatics* January: 81–83.

Kirchheimer, B. 2001. "Driving Docs to the Info Highway." Eye on Info. *Modern Healthcare* March 5 (Suppl.): 8.

Lando, M. A. 1998. "Information Technology: What Every CEO Needs to Know." *Healthcare Executive* May/June: 16–20.

Luevanos, J. 1997. "Outsourcing Cuts Operating Costs 20 Percent, Saves $1.5 Million in Capital Investment." *Health Management Technology* September: 34.

Monohan, T. 1997. "Emerging Technologies: From Fascination to Application. *Healthcare Informatics* January: 39–44.

Morrisey, J. 1998a. "Info System Evangelists." *Modern Healthcare* 28 (7): 70–85.

———. 1998b. "Data Systems' Tangible Benefits Still a Hard Sell." *Modern Healthcare* February 23: 86–90.

———. 2001a. "Slow Down: HIPAA Ahead." *Modern Healthcare* 31 (1): 30.

———. 2001b. "Crucial Support for Major Change." Eye on Info. *Modern Healthcare* March 5 (Suppl.): 18.

Ngeo, C. 1998. "A Different View of Outsourcing." *Modern Healthcare* 28 (35): 43–50.

Nussbaum, G. M. 1997. "Inside Out—The Role of the Intranet in Health Care." Published presentation, HIMSS Session 79, February. Chicago: HIMSS.

Ruffin, M. 1999. *Digital Doctors*. Tampa, FL: American College of Physician Executives.

Serb, C. 1998. "Technotravails: Computer Pros Have Seen the Future." *Hospitals & Health Networks* 72 (8): 39–40.

Shortell, S. M., et al. 2000. *Remaking Health Care in America,* 2nd edition. San Franciso: Jossey-Bass.

Solberg, C. 1998. "Gotta Have IT." *Healthcare Informatics* June: 36–38.

Solovy, A. 2000. "Is an E-Commerce Gap Emerging Among the Nation's Hospitals?" *Hospitals & Health Networks* 74 (4): 30–41.

Strassel, K. A. 1998. "Study Plays Down Internet's Economic Impact." *Wall Street Journal,* September 28, p. B9.

Tieman, J. 2001. "Dialing Up High-Tech Medicine." *Modern Healthcare* 31 (1): 36.

CHAPTER THREE

Report Cards: Competing in a Consumer-Driven Marketplace

KEY CONCEPTS: *Report cards • Consumer ratings • Patient satisfaction • Accountable markets • HEDIS data • NCQA certification • Community health information networks (CHINS)*

INTRODUCTION: In a consumer-driven marketplace, hospitals are now playing the ratings game to be a "top 100" or five-star facility. With managed care no longer a controlling factor in consumer access, many patients can choose among virtually all providers. Patient satisfaction is a critical success factor in "report card" competition. Consumer rankings provide comparative information to prospective patients searching for a hospital or doctor. Achieving "top 100 hospital" status is one of the most highly sought designations. Hospitals selected as among the best of the best can purchase the local marketing rights, splashing their national ratings on billboards and in local media. The Internet is a growing source of report card information for "med-retrievers," the online health shoppers who are looking for the best doctors, treatments, and hospitals available. Employers are also interested in steering their employees to providers with the best outcomes and lowest error rates. National databases are limited, but Medicare is working on a report card that could become a national model.

"THE INDIVIDUAL CONSUMER'S new predominance in the healthcare marketplace is increasingly influencing policy, strategy, operations and investment decisions of healthcare organizations within all segments of the industry."

—*Richard D'Amaro (1998, p. 30)*

As the United States enters the twenty-first century, the outlook for the nation's $1.3 trillion healthcare industry will be driven by population demographics and consumer behavior—not financing, managed care, health policy, government regulations, employer health benefits, new technology, or induced demand by marketing and advertising. The latter are secondary factors; they are influential, but not the ultimate driving force. To understand the future of healthcare in the new millennium, every health industry executive can be guided by a simple but profound insight—*Think customer* (Dow and Cook 1996).

As many other industries have experienced, the essence of business strategy is satisfying customers. Repeat business has the lowest marketing costs and the highest potential for word-of-mouth referrals. Healthcare is heavily dependent on consumer-to-consumer or doctor-to-consumer referrals because reliable and comparable data are not available to patients seeking the "best" hospital, doctor, or health plan. In most industries, a variety of guides have been created to assist consumers in finding high-value suppliers, defined by the factors each consumer uses to rate his or her choice—cost, reliability, or service. Valid, objective national data on healthcare organizations or health plans do not exist. But that is about to change.

Providers are becoming convinced of the impact of consumers. A national study, New Voices, on consumerism in healthcare conducted by KPMG and Northwestern University's Institute for Health Services Research and Policy Studies found that healthcare executives, physicians, and consumers themselves were strongly in agreement about "consumers' new predominance in the healthcare marketplace" (D'Amaro 1998). Anticipating the impact of the consumer revolution, healthcare executives are expecting consumers to ask more questions, demand more choices, and be more likely to complain or challenge providers. Only health plan executives in this study were less likely to support the consumerism hypothesis.

FIVE-STAR HOSPITALS: COMPETING ON THE RATINGS

Many consumers would recognize a "five-star" hotel as one of the best in the nation for service and quality. The hotel's quality would be evident by such qualities as the staff's attentive courtesy and the plush decor. But what about a "four-star" HMO or a "three-star" hospital? HealthGrades.com, based in Lakewood, Colorado, uses a five-star rating system to compare more than 3,500 hospitals. Based on Medicare data, the company makes an assessment of the relative quality of more than a dozen frequently performed hospital procedures and services (HealthGrades 2000). Another national ranking is the list of the top 100 hospitals in the United States, a highly sought rating awarded by HCIA/Sachs—the company has recently been renamed Solucient—a market research organization in Chicago. The rankings are nationally publicized in *Modern Healthcare* (Bell 2001). The company also recognizes the top 100 orthopedic hospitals and top 100 cardiovascular hospitals and provides similar rankings for stroke and intensive care units. These top-performer designations are extensively used by the winners in local marketing campaigns.

Some consumer confusion is inevitable as the first wave of consumer "report cards" attempts to provide some guidance on how to shop for a hospital, doctor, or health plan. Consumers interested to know just which are the best HMOs in the nation can simply purchase the annual guide issue. *U.S. News & World Report* also publishes an annual rating of more than 1,000 hospitals and specialty inpatient care facilities, which relies heavily on physician referral recommendations (Comarow 1997). But report cards have not yet caught on with healthcare consumers. A recent survey showed that more people (75 percent) did better research on buying cars or televisions than in shopping for the best healthcare provider (Bellandi 1998a).

To date, no national rating system or universal database is in place to make comparisons about consumer satisfaction or patient health outcomes. As mentioned earlier, *U.S. News & World* Report relies on physician referral preferences and combines those with HEDIS data from the National Committee for Quality Assurance (NCQA), which has credentialed about 50 percent of U.S. managed care plans. But not all NCQA-certified HMOs will voluntarily permit their HEDIS data to be used in comparisons such as the annual ratings issue of *U.S. News.* The plans fear that the media will not only identify the "best" HMOs but may also label lower-rated plans as "worst."

Report cards for health organizations are being produced by a number of organizations, including national news magazines, consumer publications, government health agencies, Internet health information companies, regional interest publications, business newspapers, and employer coalitions.

One of the most extensively developed healthcare guides is the product of the Southeast Michigan Employer and Purchaser Consortium, which could become a model for other regions. The 40-page guide was prepared with assistance from the Michigan Hospital Association; the Picker Institute in Boston MEDai, Inc., a health data consulting firm; and Towers Perrin, a national benefits consulting firm. Two sets of ratings were developed: *consumer satisfaction* ratings about "what patients say," and actual healthcare *outcomes,* including costs and quality. Consumers judged seven factors such as "respect for patients" and "discharge preparation," whereas outcomes focused on cost per case, complications, and length of inpatient stay. All factors, including patient satisfaction and clinical outcomes, were rated according to a three-star system:

> three stars = better than expected or than the national average;
> two stars = same as expected or at the national average;
> one star = worse than expected or than the national average.

This shoppers' guide was tough. Only one teaching hospital, the Detroit Medical Center (DMC), won an overall three-star rating from patients for medical care. Five other teaching hospitals received only one star. None of the Detroit-area hospitals, including DMC, received three-star ratings from patients in childbirth care or surgical care.

Use of the report card data is considered strictly optional, however. Employers in the area backed off from limiting their employees' choices and recommended that consumers discuss their options with their physician when selecting a hospital for their care (Southeast Michigan Employer and Purchaser Consortium 1998). No Detroit automaker or union is dictating that workers only use two star hospitals, nor are they limiting provider access in health plan networks.

SKEPTICAL CONSUMERS

A national wave of negative opinion polls and critical media have put health plans and providers on the defensive. The polls suggest that consumer confidence in health plans and providers has eroded badly. Only 15 percent of American consumers in a national study agreed completely with the statement, "I have complete confidence in hospital care," according to a poll conducted by the National Coalition on Healthcare in 1997. More than half (52 percent) of those questioned agreed completely with the statement, "There is something seriously wrong with our healthcare system." The same consumers distrusted HMOs as well, agreeing with the concern, "Quality care is often compromised by insurance companies to save money."

As this indicates, consumers are worried that their managed care plans may be more concerned with saving money than with delivering the best medical care, according to a national forecast of the healthcare marketplace prepared by VHA, based in Irving, Texas (Olson 1998, p. 49). In year 2000 election campaigns, candidates in California, North Carolina, and Texas ran successfully on anti-HMO platforms, pledging to get tough on the managed care industry and enact a "patients' bill of rights," which appears to be close to Congressional approval. Although consumers are generally more particular about service, healthcare service quality seems to be falling further in the public's esteem. In a survey conducted by *Fortune* magazine, consumers ranked healthcare services only five spots above the Internal Revenue Service in a comparison of 31 products and services (see Table 3.1).

Hospitals have a considerable consumer relations problem, according to the American Hospital Association. For the past five years, AHA has conducted a national series of consumer-focused groups and released a series of reports and videos. The AHA survey entitled "Reality Check" showcases unhappy consumers across the United States complaining that hospitals appear to be putting business interests ahead of patient care. One former patient commented, "I think there are a lot of dedicated people that work for the hospital. But the corporations that own hospitals are not humanitarian at all. They are all looking at

**Table 3.1: Consumers' Relative Satisfaction with Hospitals Versus
Other Industries**

Product or Service	Consumers' Relative Satisfaction (%)
Beverages and soft drinks	86
Long-distance phone service	81
Automobiles and trucks	79
Gasoline	77
Utilities and electric service	75
U.S. Postal Service	74
Personal computers	73
Hotels	72
Hospitals	**71**
Restaurants	70
Airlines	69
Police services	61
IRS	50

Source: Adapted from Fortune (1998).

the bottom line" (AHA 2000, p. 9). In another consumer survey sponsored by AHA, overall satisfaction with hospitals was basically high: 33 percent of Americans rated their hospital care as "excellent," and another 40 percent ranked their care as "good." Only 7 percent rated it "fair" or "poor" (AHA and Picker Institute 1998). Delving deeper into these positive findings, the Boston-based Picker Institute found that hospitals did not perform as well at providing emotional support or alleviating fears of patients (see Table 3.2).

Consumers believe that clinicians in the American health system are providing quality care, but satisfaction with the general quality of service provided in the healthcare system is mixed at best. In a consumer survey by researchers from Emery University in Atlanta, Georgia, patient satisfaction with doctors and dentists was higher than their ratings of public or nonprofit hospitals (Sheth and Mittal 1997). Consumers perceived that the "quality of cure" was often better than

Table 3.2: Patients Dissatisfied with Their Hospital Care

Patient Needs	Patients Who Reported Problems (%)
Continuity and transition	29
Emotional support	27
Information and education	24
Involvement of family/friends	24
Coordination of care	23
Respect for patient preference	22
Physical comfort	11

Source: Adapted from AHA and Picker Institute (1998, p. 4).

Table 3.3: Americans Rate Quality of Cure and Quality of Caring

Provider	Consumer Rating*
Physicians	8.47 (cure)
	8.34 (caring)
Dentists	8.66 (cure)
	8.40 (caring)
Hospitals (public)	7.86 (cure)
	7.90 (caring)
Hospitals (religious)	8.26 (cure)
	8.04 (caring)

*On a scale of 1–10, 1 being the lowest.

Source: Adapted from survey data in Sheth and Mittal (1997, p. 32).

the "quality of caring" (see Table 3.3). One in five patients would switch physicians or hospitals to get better healthcare services or products. Minority ethnic groups such as Asian Americans and Hispanic Americans were even more likely to switch providers, as were better-educated consumers versus those consumers with less education. The data reflect a relative lack of provider loyalty on the part of many consumer segments.

ARE HEALTHCARE CONSUMERS MORE SATISFIED THAN CRITICS BELIEVE?

Well-publicized studies like AHA's Reality Check have emphasized consumer concerns about the quality, accessibility, and cost of their healthcare (AHA 2000). But other household studies suggest that perhaps consumer anger is not as deep as critics have suggested. For example, KPMG/Northwestern's New Voices study found that 83 percent of Americans are "very satisfied" or "somewhat satisfied" with the quality of their care (D'Amaro 1998, p. 31). Among older adults, 82 percent of Medicare beneficiaries are satisfied. Despite widespread "HMO bashing" by critics, nearly 80 percent of all consumers polled in the KPMG/Northwestern study declared they were satisfied with the administration of their health plans.

These positive findings come at a time when HMOs are under fire in Washington, DC, and Congress is likely to enact some form of patients' bill of rights in the near future. But Washington officials should check with these employees, more than three-quarters of whom are enrolled in HMOs and who give positive ratings on health benefit coverage and plan administration.

Another study, this one of HMO members, indicates that managed care enrollees are reasonably satisfied with their health plans. The study, conducted by Hewitt & Associates, a national employee benefits firm, ranked quality, cost, and member satisfaction (Hewitt 1998). Nationally, 87 percent of the employees whose health plans were reviewed by Hewitt were satisfied with their HMOs. Some plans were rated in the 90 to 95 percent range in Pittsburgh, Pennsylvania; Toledo, Ohio; and Worcester, Massachusetts.

So are American healthcare enrollees happy, unhappy, or simply *confused*? The most accurate description may be confused, according to the first annual Health Confidence Survey by the Washington, DC–based Employee Benefit Research Institute (EBRI) (Cochrane 1998). Although 83 percent of people covered by commercial health insurance are in some form of managed care plan, 56 percent of the managed care enrollees in the EBRI study say they have "never been covered under a managed care plan." A majority of those who label their current plan as an HMO, preferred provider organization (PPO), or point-of-service (POS) plan, also say "they have never been in managed care." Healthcare consumers, then, appear to be confused about what managed care is. Their inability to define managed care brings into question findings such as "those who are enrolled in private, non–managed care plans are more satisfied—71 percent versus 57 percent—in comparison with managed care participants." EBRI officials found participants in their Health Confidence Survey to be "massively confused" about what type of insurance they actually have, casting some doubt on the findings in their studies and others that were critical of managed care.

THE BABY BOOMERS ARE COMING ... AND ARE THEY DEMANDING!

As the baby boom generation pulls the United States into the new millennium, the country's population of 270 million will experience mushrooming growth over the next 25 years. Some 75 million boomers—one-third of the total U.S. population—will be reaching age 65 in the year 2011. They are the largest single segment of consumers, but numerous other changes will also occur in America's demographics between now and the year 2020.

The Bureau of the Census projects demographic growth and change as follows (U.S. Bureau of the Census 1998):

- Total population will soar from 270 million to up to 322 million Americans—an increase of almost 20 percent.
- The gender gap will continue, with men comprising 48.9 percent and women 51.1 percent of the population in the year 2020.
- Ethnic groups will grow at least twice as fast as the white population, including blacks (+30.5 percent), American Indians (+33.9 percent), and Asian/Pacific Islanders (+87.5 percent).
- The senior population over age 65 will more than double (+56.0 percent), to more than 50 million.

The baby boom generation could be the most demanding health-care consumers ever. A national study by the South Bend, Indiana–based Press-Ganey research organization reported that people born between 1946 and 1964 are much less satisfied with the quality of their healthcare services than are older generations (Bellandi 1998b). Analysis of data from more than one million patients showed a consistent pattern—older patients gave higher marks to every aspect of healthcare from quality of food to cheerfulness of the hospital. Baby boomers were less often satisfied and more likely to be critical, according to the study, which analyzed patient satisfaction with both hospital and home care services.

THE ERA OF ACCOUNTABILITY IS ARRIVING

Although based on crude and limited data, report cards on healthcare providers are now becoming available. As implied by the discussion in chapter 2, the healthcare system is in the middle of a profound revolution toward accountability, predicts Don Berwick, M.D., of the Boston-based Institute for Healthcare Improvement (Berwick 1997). Berwick believes a fundamental change will occur in America's $1.3 trillion health system. Competition on quality and outcomes will replace price as the leading factor in purchasing decisions by employers and consumers. Berwick foresees accountable markets will "gather enough information on performance, use enough good tools, and report the findings to the payers and the public" (Berwick 1997, p. 246). If this scenario works, healthcare will improve through the "invisible hand" of competition. Some observers are skeptical about the impact of such reports, and the skeptics could be right. Online national databases like HealthGrades.com have become available in the past three years to compare provider or plan performance, but whether many consumers are using the information is not clear. An indication may lie in the fact that, in early 2001, HealthGrades.com was in danger of being delisted by the NASDAQ stock exchange because its stock price had slipped below the NASDAQ minimum of $1 per share.

National ratings for HMOS are among the first report cards to become available to consumers. *U.S. News & World Report*'s cover story,

"Best HMOS: America's Most Complete Guide," is a case in point. As mentioned in chapter 2, the report profiles the best HMOS in every state, but the report is far from comprehensive. Hundreds of America's 650 HMOS did not participate because they were not rated by NCQA. Dozens of other plans are not listed because they consider media use of NCQA data to be unsophisticated or unfair. Some 149 managed care plans refused to make their HEDIS data available to *U.S. News'* reporters this year. One national HMO objected to the way the media have used NCQA data in the past. "It was your report in *U.S. News* that triggered the decision" not to participate, according to the plan's chief medical officer (Comarow 1998, p. 77).

Employer demands for a national rating system for HMOS has spurred the growth of NCQA, based in Washington, DC. About half of the 650 licensed HMOS are participating in its credentialing program and are surveyed every three years against a comprehensive set of standards. The NCQA requires that all managed care plans conduct an annual random "core sample" of 1,800 enrollees to determine member satisfaction with the plan.

Enrollee satisfaction data would be even more useful if the plans would obtain consumer ratings each year from the same members to track consumer ratings over time. Several large corporations, including Xerox and GTE, conduct a periodic enrollee satisfaction study, comparing plan members' responses to 154 questions in two studies conducted at two-year intervals (Allen and Rogers 1997). Some 21 HMOS were rated in the surveys. Researchers deliberately oversampled people more likely to be sick to balance the substantially larger group of healthy enrollees who make only limited use of the health plans. The results showed that independent practice associations (IPAS) were the most popular form of health plan but were only marginally better rated than prepaid group practice or POS plans (see Table 3.4). Some changes occurred over time. IPAS were not as highly rated in the second survey, whereas indemnity, which had the lowest rating in the first survey, soared to the most popular model in the follow-up survey. Researchers also found that enrollees who had switched plans between surveys were much less satisfied with their plans than "stayers," those who did not change plans. Indemnity plan members were the most likely to

Table 3.4: Consumer Satisfaction with HMOs: A Longitudinal Study (1993 and 1995)—Overall Plan Satisfaction

Plan Type	1993	1995	Change
IPA	86.4	83.4	−3.0
Prepaid group practice	84.2	84.0	−0.2
POS	74.6	72.6	−2.0
Indemnity	69.9	85.0	+15.1

Source: Adapted from Allen and Rogers (1997, p. 160).

change plan models. Overall, ratings dropped from the first survey to the second.

DEFINING A NATIONAL STANDARD

If Medicare adopts a report card, it could become a universal model for other payers and purchasers. In Washington, DC, the Agency for Healthcare Research and Quality (AHRQ) (formerly known as the Agency for Health Care Policy and Research) is developing a satisfaction survey for all Medicare-risk health plans (Grimaldi 1997). The survey is based in part on HEDIS 3.0, developed by NCQA. Medicare's satisfaction survey is being developed as part of the Consumer Assessment of Health Plans (CAHPS®) study. A draft of the survey has been in the works for three years but is still undergoing testing and is not yet ready for consideration as federal regulation.

Medicare is basing its report card development on the NCQA HEDIS model. HCFA has, in fact, contracted with NCQA to develop and refine a "HEDIS-type" survey for Medicare HMOs. The current HEDIS 3.0 survey asks 39 questions; Medicare's draft HMO survey asks 61 questions. Many of the questions are the same as in the HEDIS 3.0 questionnaire, but even minor differences between the two surveys will make comparison of their HMO enrollees' satisfaction with commercial HMO members more difficult. Questions included in the draft Medicare HMO survey ask patients if they:

- had trouble making appointments;
- were not referred for specialist care desired;
- felt discharged too soon if hospitalized;
- used some home health care but wanted more;
- felt home health care was needed but did not receive it;
- were able to see the same physician for most scheduled visits;
- would rate highly the overall quality of healthcare covered by plan; and
- would recommend plan to family or friends.

Enrollee satisfaction findings for Medicare HMO members will probably be compared to similar survey data for Medicare fee-for-service beneficiaries. HCFA now conducts an annual "Medicare Current Beneficiary Study," a longitudinal survey of about 12,000 seniors. HCFA collects information on their healthcare utilization as well as satisfaction with access and service quality. Progress on a Medicare HMO enrollee survey was slowed by HCFA's Y2K computer system problems; thus, its launch still has not been implemented.

NATIONAL REPORT CARDS WILL NEED NATIONAL DATABASES

Many potholes still appear on the information highway. National report cards will need national databases, which exist only in fragments in the health field. Paul Starr, author of *The Social Transformation of American Medicine*, laments, "There is no industry giant, like Microsoft, to drive the health industry towards standardization and cost efficiency" (Starr 1998, p. 91). Computer networks providing comparable data could raise the quality of care and provide a new basis for competition on outcomes and patient satisfaction. But lack of cooperation between government agencies and many segments of the health industry have frustrated efforts to resolve key issues around standards and access.

Disputes in Congress between liberals and conservatives over the role of government have delayed bipartisan cooperation on health data issues. Both Democrats and Republicans have demonized the data issue. The GOP has largely blocked efforts at expanding health data networks, raising concerns about privacy and expansion of government. More liberal Democrats have viewed health data as an opportunity to advance the cause of national health reform. Congress may enact a patients' bill of rights in 2001, but given the current balance of power between Democrats and Republicans, the chances for enactment of a national health information database appear limited.

Many issues are yet to be overcome before national report cards for the health industry could become available.

- *Cost*—Even with bipartisan support from Congress, health networks would still have to overcome issues of cost and who would pay.
- *Universal connectivity*—The rise of the Internet offers a new opportunity to build national health data networks that could provide a universal, current database for healthcare report cards.
- *Public and private database linkages*—Internet connections could provide the linkages between public databases such as those from Medicare cost reports and private data such as health insurers and HMOs.
- *Universal patient identifier*—One of the many issues to be overcome would be establishing a universal patient identifier, for example, social security number, which would require government action and broad industry cooperation.
- *Definitions and standards*—The health sector has lagged in adopting common data definitions ("data dictionaries") and standards for electronic data interchange.
- *Hardware and software*—Hospitals are now well connected in Internet-based networks, but numerous physician offices and other care settings must still become Internet equipped.

- *Voluminous data and multiple providers*—Few industries can match healthcare for the heavy volume of data that is supplied by multiple, disconnected providers.

Voluntary local initiatives to build health data networks have generally failed. The Hartford Foundation provided substantial grant funding to seven community health management information systems (CHMISS) in the early 1990s. Five statewide CHMIS projects were launched, plus regional projects in New York City and Memphis. Ultimately, the complexity of technical and political issues overwhelmed these voluntary activities, even with strong community support and outside funding.

Other local efforts to launch cooperative data networks, called community health information networks (CHINS) in Milwaukee, Wisconsin, and in Utah have had some limited success, but a similar effort in Chicago failed. In California, a large-scale CHIN project involving 40 public and private organizations is now providing information exchange services, claims transmission, and eligibility verification for more than half of insured Californians. The California project is more like an "enterprise network" that provides a defined business function on behalf of one or more strategic business partners. Experience with CHINS and the CHMIS pilot projects suggests that future data networks are more likely to be successful if they are established for clear, limited business purposes in proprietary arrangements.

National policy has still not resolved the two key issues regarding computerized health information: how to keep private what ought to be private, and how to make public what should be public (Starr 1998, p. 103). Congress mandated national standards for health data privacy, giving the secretary of the Department of Health and Human Services the power to implement data standards if Congress does not act to adopt them. But concerns about electronic medical records and privacy have now become wrapped up with the consumer protection debate and competing proposals for a patient bill of rights. Regardless of that outcome, the incremental establishment of national health information databases is likely in the next three to five years, starting with the pending Medicare HEDIS-type report card on enrollee satisfaction and health promotion activities. The era of healthcare report cards will soon be arriving.

TEN ACTION STEPS TO A CONSUMER-DRIVEN MARKETPLACE

Numerous hospitals and health systems are scrambling to catch up with the consumer movement. Some consultants recommend that establishing a patient-centered culture is essential, where care workers stop referring to "patients" and start calling them "customers." Patient satisfaction consultant K. C. Warner of Press-Ganey in South Bend, Indiana, asks: "But is that consistent with the health organization's culture? You have instituted a customer service program. You are collecting survey data. Do you still feel like things are not going the way you wanted them to? Do you feel like there is a mixture of cultures at work in your facility that may not support patient satisfaction?" (Warner 1998, p. 1).

Physicians and nurses may react negatively to "consumerism" in healthcare, if it means a business orientation as opposed to a focus on putting patients first. Physicians are coming to understand that the "functional quality" of the doctor-patient interaction—patients' perceptions of their care—can be as important as the technical quality of medical science (Bradley 2001, p. 6). Not everyone in the community believes that their nonprofit hospital's motto really is, "We'll take care of you regardless of your ability to pay," and trustees are shocked to learn this (Wright 1997, p. 22).

Plan now for the report card era. Evaluate programs for patient satisfaction. Survey access and service perceptions of the community. Learn what local employers think of healthcare quality and costs. Allow physicians and employees to report candidly about quality and service issues. Get used to living under a media microscope. The defining moment for becoming patient centered is different in every organization. Creating a customer orientation must continue to reflect the traditions, values, and "way things get done around here."

Ten action steps to become customer focused follow.

1. Use Patient Satisfaction Surveys

A new generation of patient satisfaction measuring tools is being developed by organizations such as Press-Ganey in South Bend, Indiana, and the Picker Institute in Boston. Picker is participating in CAHPS® with AHRQ, (Edgman-Levitan and Gertels 1998), and HCFA is working with NCQA to develop the HEDIS-type report card for the Medicare program.

Press-Ganey, a leading consumer satisfaction rating organization, has the largest customer base among U.S. hospitals. Its research instruments cover more than a dozen settings, many of them ambulatory. In 1999, Press-Ganey introduced a new Medical Practice questionnaire, which triggered a phenomenal 300 percent growth rate in the number of facilities that want to evaluate patient satisfaction in doctors' offices (Drain 2001). More than 1,000 medical practices now use the instrument. Results of the questionnaire indicate that average satisfaction is rated at 86.6, midway between "good" (75) and "very good" (100). Managed care may play a role in patients' satisfaction with their physicians, where shorter visits and less time for questions are often observed. Doctors in the western United States had the lowest average satisfaction ratings (82.3), and the highest were registered in New England (89.2), where managed care is not as well established.

2. Compile Dashboard Indicators of Quality

Governance consultant Jamie Orlikoff, based in Oak Brook, Illinois, recommends that provider organizations compile and regularly assess a limited set of quality indicators as they monitor financial performance. These dashboard indicators would provide an ongoing surveillance system for key factors such as consumer satisfaction and clinical outcomes. Other factors should be evaluated yearly, such as employee turnover, physician referrals, and other benchmarks of the organizational climate. Paying regular attention at the board level to service and quality, as well as finances, will send a message to the organization about priorities and putting patients first.

3. Establish Toll-Free Consumer Hot Lines

A growing number of hospitals and health systems have established consumer "call centers" to provide advice and information to consumers. Call centers can be shared by a number of hospitals or physician organizations on a regional or even multimarket basis. National call center providers include Access Health, a division of McKesson/HBOC, whose "Ask A Nurse" call centers were early models for consumer information and marketing. Call centers use standardized protocols and are staffed by nurses and other trained specialists who handle both clinical and service access questions. Many HMOs have also established toll-free consumer call centers to provide "access management" referrals and health plan information.

4. Initiate Consumer Focus Groups

Structured and facilitated focus groups can provide an in-depth perspective on consumer attitudes and values, which will supplement and enrich report card data. Consumer participation in focus groups can provide context to testing of consumer issues and preferences, and computer polling can provide quantitative data to focus groups, in addition to videotaping and note taking. For example, in Minneapolis, Professional Feedback Systems provides a number of computer-based interactive market research services (Bennett-Leet 1998).

Using keypads, laptops, and specialized software, consumer focus groups go high-tech with the following tools.

- Audience surveys on specialized diskettes creatively use questions to challenge, inform, and stimulate thinking. Surveys can be issued in advance, concurrently, or post-session using e-mail and web sites.
- On-site research using interactive polling technology can ask pre-established questions, as well as quickly incorporate brainstorming, group discussion, and refined issues.
- Priority setting technology allows consumers to rate, rank, and compare any issue, statement, or product. Consumer preferences

can be identified by consumer subgroups easily but without disclosing identities.

- Team or group comparisons can be compiled using computer polling technology. Consumer preferences can be evaluated over time, as well as across geographic areas or consumer subgroups.

5. Benchmark Organizational Performance

A growing number of hospitals and healthcare service programs are evaluating their experience with those of comparable organizations. The Solucient (formerly HCIA/Sachs) top 100 hospitals provide benchmarks for the field and encourage high performance across the industry. The company is publicly sharing some detailed benchmarks in areas such as pediatric length of stay, breast cancer management, and coronary angioplasties (Bell 2001). For instance, in orthopedics, the top 100 study found that all winning hospitals had 3.5 percent lower severity- and wage-adjusted costs, compared to peers. Their patient satisfaction scores were in the top percentile of rankings, and economic costs were in the top quartile.

Many hospitals have ongoing patient satisfaction research programs on a year-round basis. Press-Ganey, as mentioned, has more than 1,000 clients. Other national organizations such as the Picker Institute and Solucient provide extensive comparison data. Press-Ganey consultant Mary Malone (1998) argues, "Since healthcare's historical approach to providing information, explanations, and education has been to withhold information, this is an area where we have tremendous opportunity to make a positive impact."

6. Link Management Compensation to Consumer Satisfaction Ratings

A powerful reinforcing link can be built between report card data and management compensation. Managers' performance assessment tools can incorporate quantitative goals and benchmarks for service quality. Every manager would incorporate service quality indicators into his or her performance goals and assess progress on a periodic and annual basis. Special bonuses for quality could be structured on a monthly or quarterly basis. These can be established for managerial performance as well as for operating units, which each have their own service quality goals.

7. Conduct Local Consumer Surveys

National studies are no substitute for local data on consumer perceptions. Local consumer studies can be conducted by professional marketing consulting firms or by internal planning and marketing staff. Some hospitals have experimented with using trustees to conduct their own "on the street" surveys with people in the community, asking them a limited number of questions, such as the following (Wright 1997):

- Do you think the number of uninsured persons in our community is going up or down?
- Would an uninsured person believe that hospital or emergency care is available to everyone without regard to pay?
- Is the quality of healthcare in the community going up, staying the same, or getting worse?

8. Hire Patient Advocates

A growing number of hospitals and health systems are employing patient advocates. Hiring patient advocates formalizes their consumer service orientation and provides an ongoing administrative focus for continuously improving patient service. Patient advocates can provide a link between patients and their families and the staff caregivers and institution to improve communications and solve problems. In recent labor negotiations, the Kaiser Health System agreed with the California Nursing Association to establish 18 patient advocate positions within the multihospital Kaiser system. Patient advocates can continuously monitor service quality data provided by external firms such as Press-Ganey and the Picker Institute, as well as data from the organization's internal management information system.

9. Create Web Sites and Interactive Web Pages

The Internet is transforming healthcare into a hands-on affair for patients. With just a few mouse clicks, consumers are increasingly accessing a trove of medical journals, support groups, and medical advice providers, creating a market trend that has been noted in the *Wall Street Journal* (Quick 1998). As more consumers obtain access to the Internet, providers can use the Web to survey consumer attitudes and measure how patients and the community rate their services. Mainstream Web-based health information providers include the Mayo Clinic, Johns Hopkins, and the National Library of Medicine. In a recent study of consumers on the Web, Jupiter Communications estimated that 30 million "med-retrievers"—online health information consumers—went to the Internet for health information (Flory 2001). These consumers tend to be older, female, and ethnically diverse. Med-retrievers are also educated, with at least one year of college, and they are affluent, with a projected annual household income of at least $80,000. Increased sophistication on the part of users is driving Web content providers to upgrade the depth of their information and to add content on alternative medicine.

10. Promote Community Education and Marketing

Direct-to-consumer marketing by pharmaceutical firms is part of a wider trend to reach consumers by informing them. Competing on service ratings and report card data will become commonplace in the new millennium. Already, hospitals that have been highly rated in reports such as *U.S. News*' "Best Hospitals in America" are splashing their ratings in mass-media marketing and public education. More than a few top-ranked institutions are trumpeting their ratings on billboards and full-page news advertisements. Several ratings organizations charge hospitals marketing fees for use of the ratings and, in some cases, sell "franchise protection" against a rival that might also be highly ranked. Health plans are conducting expensive multimedia advertising campaigns based on their *U.S. News* rankings as well as on

HEDIS data. Some health plans and provider organizations are using their own commissioned market research studies to identify those hospitals or specialized care programs that are most widely recognized as "number one" by local consumers. As report cards become widely available, heavy competition in the ratings game should be expected.

In trendy Southern California, the five-hospital Memorial Health System of Long Beach, which is branded under the name Memorial-Care, is engaging in outcomes-based marketing. Few provider organizations have done what MemorialCare is doing—providing specific clinical outcomes on its web site (Hagland 2001). MemorialCare's web site publishes a quality report card that reports clinical outcome data in six patient care areas: angina, breast care, cardiac care, hip and knee procedures, obstetric care, and complications. For example, Memorial-Care's angina survival rate is 98.8 percent, compared with 96.2 percent for all California hospitals and 95.4 percent for hospitals nationwide. The outcomes campaign is based on the system's decision to brand itself around a total commitment to quality. Despite the potential for controversy, MemorialCare believes it is receiving a very positive response from consumers and physicians. It has also strengthened the system's position in managed care contracting. Outcomes-based marketing is a high-value strategy for the millennium marketplace.

LOOKING FORWARD: WILL HEALTHCARE CONSUMERS ACTUALLY USE REPORT CARDS?

A fundamental question is still to be answered: Will healthcare consumers actually use report cards? Research studies show that consumers want cost and access information about health plans and providers but are less interested in consumer satisfaction or independent ratings by experts. A study by the Kaiser Family Foundation found that only 39 percent of consumers had information comparing health plans, and less than one-third of that group said they used this information themselves (Robinson and Brodie 1997). In Massachusetts, more than 3,000 government employees, retirees, and their dependents rated the information that the consumers considered most essential (see Table 3.5). The two lowest-ranked items were "percentage of persons who are

Table 3.5: Information that Consumers Rate as "Essential"

Type of Information	Rating (%)
Specific benefits	72.0
Average out-of-pocket costs	61.7
Quality of primary care physicians	53.7
Premium prices	51.6
Quality of specialty physicians	47.5
Convenience of obtaining referrals	45.3
Quality of preventive care	43.1
Convenience of seeing primary care physician	32.2
Convenience of paperwork	20.9
Quality of mental health and substance abuse care	19.1
Satisfaction with plan	18.4
Ratings of plan by experts	17.1

Source: Adapted from Tumlinson et al. (1997).

satisfied with the plan overall" (member satisfaction) and "ratings of each plan by independent experts" (report cards) (Tumlinson et al. 1997).

With Medicare, employers, and NCQA lined up to produce report cards, then, a preliminary answer to our question comes from the Pennsylvania Healthcare Cost Containment Council. The Council has produced an annual report on open-heart surgery, the Consumer Guide to Coronary Artery Bypass Graft (CABG) Surgery, since 1992. A state agency, the Council has been at the forefront of efforts to inform consumers about cardiac surgery, based on reliable, risk-adjusted data on every Pennsylvania hospital, surgeon, and surgical group providing CABG surgery. The agency produced and distributed 15,000 copies of the first two yearly surveys and continues to receive widespread media coverage when the updated report, covering 41 heart surgery programs in the Keystone State, is issued.

If Pennsylvania's experience is any illustration, the strategy of informing consumers still falls well below the mark in affecting patient choice. According to a recent study in the *Journal of the American*

Medical Association (JAMA), only 12 percent of patients who actually received CABG surgery were aware of the state's report card on cardiac mortality before undergoing heart surgery (Schneider and Epstein 1998). Fewer than one percent of these open-heart surgery patients knew the correct rating of their hospital or surgeon or claimed that the report card had influenced their choice of provider. The dismaying statistics on the ineffectiveness of report cards provide a strong indication of how to tailor an extensive consumer education campaign if report cards are to have much impact.

Report cards on the performance of hospitals, doctors, or health plans all have the same intent—to help healthcare consumers make more informed choices. Well-regarded ratings exist in a number of other fields, such as J. D. Power's consumer satisfaction ratings of new automobiles. But healthcare has no similar tradition or database. As report cards appear, providers and plans will predictably develop advertising and marketing campaigns that extract data that puts their organizations in the best light. The *JAMA* study showed that open-heart surgery patients had to make a choice within three days of getting word that they were undergoing surgery; thus the window of opportunity to influence consumer choice is limited. Realistically, the backers of report cards need to take a number of steps to make comparative market data more effective to influence consumer behavior:

- Extensive consumer education is essential for consumers to become aware that comparative information is available.
- Report card data must be widely accessible to potential consumers, using an array of communications media.
- Physician support is essential, for example, making report cards available in waiting rooms, because many consumers will seek information at the point of service.
- Current data are more likely to be trusted by consumers, even if older data may be gathered in a more statistically valid way.
- The Internet is rapidly becoming a primary channel for report card data. Online patient support groups will become channels for transmitting and interpreting report card information.

- Media can rapidly broaden the availability of report card data and should be considered partners in the consumer education process.
- Report card information must be available on a timely basis, within days after diagnosis, if consumers are to benefit in making informed choices.

The accountability revolution will take place in the near future as report cards become widely available in the next three to five years. Consumers will have access to data on medical performance once considered highly confidential. Skeptics will question whether more than a handful of consumers will actually obtain or rely on report cards when selecting providers or plans, but Dr. Donald Berwick raises a more fundamental concern: any company that confines its view of customer-mindedness to the report cards and ratings currently absorbing so much time and energy would rapidly go out of business. Such companies would "waste far too much energy on looking better and not enough on becoming better" (Berwick 1997).

STRATEGIC IMPLICATIONS

The ratings wars are on. Employers want accountability; consumers want information; providers want a competitive advantage. A whole new marketplace is taking shape.

Assume Smart Consumers. Report cards will change the playing field. Prepare for informed consumers. Armed with Internet-based information and provider-to-provider comparisons, consumers now stand on near-equal footing with their doctors in selecting their care sources and sites.

Quality Becomes the Number One Competitive Factor. Competing on quality and customer satisfaction—not cost—will reinvent the marketplace. Every hospital and doctor will now fear medical errors. Report cards and public data on performance will stimulate a higher emphasis on clinical outcomes. Cost data still motivate health plans, but the plans cannot afford to ignore the top-rated facilities in the market.

Compete to Be Best of the Best. Benchmarking organizational performance with the best in the nation is the challenge for every management team, board of trustees, and medical staff. Data on clinical outcomes, lengths of stay, and other key performance parameters will be public. Those who succeed in improving their performance—and their report card ratings—will boost their market reputation and market share.

REFERENCES

Allen, H. M., and W. H. Rogers. 1997. "The Consumer Health Plan Value Survey: Round Two." *Health Affairs* 16 (4): 156–66.

American Hospital Association (AHA). 2000. *Reality Check III: Searching for Trust,* pp. 1–25. Chicago: AHA.

American Hospital Association (AHA) and the Picker Institute. 1998. "Eye on Patients: Excerpts from a Report on Patients' Concerns and Experiences About the Healthcare System." *Hospitals & Health Networks* 23 (4): 2–11.

Bell, C. 2001. "100 Top Hospitals: National Benchmarks." *Modern Healthcare* 31 (8, Special Suppl.): 1–40.

Bellandi, D. 1998a. "Consumers First." *Modern Healthcare* 28 (4): 30–31.

———. 1998b. "Healthcare Not Satisfying Boomers." *Modern Healthcare* 28 (4): 30.

Bennett-Leet, D. 1998. "Interactive Programs: The People Side of Change," pp. 1–4. Minneapolis, MN: Professional Feedback Systems.

Berwick, D. M. 1997. "The Total Customer Relationship in Healthcare: Broadening the Bandwith." *Journal on Quality Improvement* 23 (5): 245–50.

Bradley, W. J. 2001. "Patient Satisfaction: Not a New Era of Healthcare." *The Satisfaction Monitor,* pp. 6–7. South Bend, IN: Press-Ganey.

Cochrane, J. 1998. "What Consumer Backlash?" *Integrated Healthcare Report* 5 (4): 3–11.

Comarow, A. 1997. America's Best Hospitals. *U.S. News & World* Report: 1–508.

———. 1998. "Plans That Opted Out." *U.S. News & World Report* 125 (13): 77–78.

D'Amaro, R. 1998. "Consumers' Increasing Influence on Healthcare." *Caring* June: 30–31.

Dow, R., and S. Cook. 1996. *Turned On: Eight Vital Insights to Energize Your People, Customers and Profits.* New York: Harper Business.

Drain, R. 2001. "Medical Practice Questionnaire Provides New Data on Physician Offices." *The Satisfaction Monitor,* January, pp. 3–4.

Edgman-Levitan, S., and M. Gertels. 1998. "Measures of Quality: What Can Public Reporting Accomplish?" *Healthcare Forum Journal* January/February: 27, 36–37.

Flory, J. 2001. "Consumer Expectations to Reshape Providers' Net Strategies." *Internet Healthcare Strategies* 3 (3): 10–11.

Fortune. 1998. "Americans Are More Finicky than Ever: Industries Ranked from Best to Worst." *Fortune* 35 (2): 108–10.

Grimaldi, P. L. 1997. "Are Managed Care Members Satisfied?" *Nursing Management* 28 (6): 12–15.

Hagland, M. 2001. "Effective Marketing with Clincal Outcomes Data." COR *Healthcare Market Strategist* 2 (3): 1, 11–14.

HealthGrades. 2000. "Hospital Report Cards Methodology White Paper: 2001 Analysis" (1997–1999 data), August 22, pp. 1–3. Lakewood, CO: HealthGrades.

Hewitt & Associates. 1998. "Hewitt Health Value Initiative." Cited in Cochrane, J. 1998. "What Consumer Backlash?" *Integrated Healthcare Report* 5 (4): 8–11.

Malone, M. P. 1998. "What Do Patients Want to Know and When Do They Want to Know It?" *The Satisfaction Monitor* 15 (3): 11.

National Coalition on Healthcare. 1997. "How Americans Perceive the Health-care System: A Report of a National Survey." *Journal of Healthcare Finance* 23 (4): 12–20.

Olson, M. I. 1998. *Environmental Assessment: Setting Foundations for the Millennium,* pp. 1–174. Irving, TX: VHA Inc.

Quick, R. 1998. "Click Here." *Wall Street Journal,* October 19, p. R10.

Robinson, S., and M. Brodie. 1997. "Understanding the Quality Challenge for Health Consumers: The Kaiser/AHCPR Survey." *Journal on Quality Improvement* 23 (5): 239–244.

Schneider, E. C., and A. M. Epstein. 1998. "Use of Public Performance Reports." *Journal of the American Medical Association* 279 (20): 1638–42.

Sheth, J. N., and B. Mittal. 1997. "The Health of the Healthcare Industry: A Report from American Consumers." *Marketing Health Services* 17 (4): 29–35.

Southeast Michigan Employer and Purchaser Consortium. 1998. *Southeast Michigan Hospital Performance Profile: A Consumer Guide,* pp. 1–42. Detroit, MI: Southeast Michigan Employer and Purchaser Consortium.

Starr, P. 1998. "Smart Technology, Stunted Policy: Developing Health Information Networks." *Health Affairs* 16 (3): 91–105.

Tumlinson, A., H. Bottigheimer, P. Mahoney, M. Elliot, and A. Hendricks. 1997. "Choosing A Health Plan: What Information Will Consumers Use?" *Health Affairs* 16 (3): 229–38.

U.S. Bureau of the Census. 1998. "Population Projections of the United States, by Age, Sex, Race, and Hispanic Origin, 1995 to 2050." Current Population Reports, pp. 98–103. Washington, DC: Government Printing Office [Cited in *Universal Health Almanac.*]

Warner, K. C. 1998. "Leading a Patient Centered Care Culture." *The Satisfaction Monitor* 15 (2): 1–2.

Wright, A. P. 1997. "Perception is Reality." *Trustee* 50 (4): 22–24.

CHAPTER FOUR

Connecting Businesses

KEY CONCEPTS: *B2B* • *Disintermediation* • *Internet commerce* • *Online medical buying* • *Internet speed* • *Strategic e-relationships*

INTRODUCTION: The hoped-for "killer application" of the World Wide Web is "B2B"—business-to-business. Participants include Fortune 500 companies, health product "e-tailers" and online B2B exchanges, small start-up companies, and Internet entrepreneurs like medibuy and Neoforma. Healthcare organizations are restructuring and disintermediating in the $1.3 trillion industry, looking for savings in the estimated $150 billion of health expenditures which are administrative waste. Healthcare Internet commerce could reach $370 billion by 2004, according to Forrester Research. Migrating many of healthcare's business processes to the Internet offers great promise; better business solutions, lower prices, and customized processes and products are all possible. Online medical buying could save 15 to 20 percent, with lowest-cost transaction costs, product standardization, adherence to contract compliance, and enterprise best practices. As hundreds of digital e-marketplaces continue to roll out at "Internet speed," e-commerce experts predict that only two to three Internet companies will survive and become profitable in each industry before burning through their venture capital. The battle for control of e-commerce in healthcare is already forcing rapid consolidation, and the e-newcomers are forming strategic relationships with traditional wholesalers, group purchasing organizations, and distributors.

"EVERY BUSINESS IS an information business .... About one-third of the cost of health care in the United States—some $350 billion— consists of the cost of capturing, storing, processing, and retrieving information: patient records, cost accounting and insurance claims. By that measure, health care is a larger information industry than the 'information industry.' "

—*Philip Evans and Thomas Wurster (2000, p. 9)*

Internet advocates believe that business-to-business (b2b) enterprise will be the ultimate "killer application" of the World Wide Web (Coile 2000). Participants include Fortune 500 companies, health product electronic retailers ("e-tailers"), online b2b exchanges, small start-up companies, and Internet entrepreneurs like medibuy and Neoforma. Healthcare organizations are restructuring and disintermediating in the $1.3 trillion industry, looking for savings in the estimated $350 billion of health expenditures that are administrative waste (Halter 2000). Healthcare Internet commerce could reach $370 billion by 2004, according to Forrester Research (see Table 4.1), which monitors Web trends and electronic commerce (Meyer 2000a).

Transforming commerce in healthcare is proving a tough sell, at least at this time. The story of Healtheon/WebMD is a cautionary tale of bold visions and mega-investments in healthcare e-commerce that so far have failed to approach the founders'—or the investors'—original expectations (Carrns 2001). In the mid-1990s, Internet pioneer Jim Clark, founder of Netscape, had a grand vision to focus on a $350 billion dollar target—administrative waste in healthcare—by removing half of the excess overhead in the health industry. He founded Healtheon to replace person-to-person interchanges like physician billings with Internet-automated, b2b exchanges at a fraction of the costs (Lewis 2000). Clark built Healtheon from an Internet start-up in 1998 into a sizeable company by purchasing Envoy, Medical Manager, CareInsite, and more than a dozen other companies. Clark's belief was that Healtheon "could be as big as Microsoft, and quicker, too" (Lewis 2000). The company's aggressive, multibillion dollar acquisition strategy of medical management and electronic claims processing firms included increasing its potential to challenge HMOs and

Table 4.1: E-Health Market Forecast, 1999–2004 ($ in Billions)

Year	E-Health B2B	E-Health B2C	Total Internet E-Health
1999	$ 6	$ 0.4	$ 6.4
2002	81	6.0	87.0
2004	348	22.0	370.0

Source: Forrester Research, "Sizing Healthcare E-Commerce," cited in Halter (2000, p. 122).

established third-party intermediaries like EDS and many Blue Cross plans. Clark merged Healtheon with Atlanta-based WebMD in early 1999 in a $4.8 billion deal, which gave the company access to 400,000 physician desktops. Managing the new firm, Healtheon/WebMD, was Jeffrey Arnold, the 31-year-old entrepreneur who leveraged a great brand name, WebMD, and $250 million investment by Microsoft into one of the health industry's largest Internet-based companies. Two years later, Arnold was out of the firm and Medco founder Martin Wygood had taken over, quickly slashing 20 percent of the staff and consolidating in New Jersey the company's many acquired companies. Wygood has scaled back the company's business plan to focus on a more modest goal: selling software and services, primarily insurance claims, and other forms of transaction processing to health plans and doctors.

The slowdown of the dot-com sector cast a chill over electronic commerce applications in healthcare. Whereas other sectors of the economy are transforming their businesses with information technology and the Internet, healthcare organizations are more reluctant to commit to Internet-enabled solutions. Despite a 47 percent increase in e-commerce software spending by hospitals in the first six months of 2000, a recent poll of healthcare executives for AHA discovered the presence of "e-skepticism" (Coile 2001). Only 43 percent of the *Futurescan* survey panel believe that the Internet would significantly reduce costs for purchasers of healthcare supplies and equipment, a significant drop from the 76 percent support rating from last year's survey.

REDEFINING BUSINESS

The Internet is redefining business in every sector, from entertainment to transportation. What distinguishes the new economy from that of the past is the shift in power from producers to consumers. Consumers demand, and expect to get, the best quality and service at the lowest prices. They want it customized, and they want it immediately (Sculley and Woods 1999). Any development that reduces overhead is a winner, and the Internet should do just that. Indeed, a new set of strategies is being developed for health and medical products to capitalize on this new efficient marketplace. The Amazon.com model turned bookselling on its head, not simply because of its increased customer reach via low-cost Internet access, but also and primarily because of the attendant reduction of overhead costs. Internet consultant Bill Gross of Cleveland-based Medimetrex likes Amazon.com because the entire company runs on the same number of full-time employees (FTES) as run one Barnes and Noble bookstore (Gross 2000).

The competition is no longer between large and small firms, but between fast and slow. Change is happening in Internet time, fast and furious. The first companies to attract significant market attention were business-to-consumer (B2C) firms, like Amazon.com and drkoop .com. But market momentum is shifting to B2B. Industry analysts predict that business-to-business Internet companies will be many times larger than B2C enterprises. Three years after emerging into the spotlight, the Internet poses a difficult challenge for established businesses, which over time have carefully built brands and physical distribution relationships. These could all be destroyed by the new economy's Internet-based opportunities for establishing new channels to consumers, distributors, and suppliers while reducing costs by eliminating many of the third parties in the process (Evans and Wurster 2000).

B2B IN HEALTHCARE

Electronic commerce in healthcare is progressing but is not yet moving at Internet speed. The healthcare industry has not embraced the Internet as quickly as other sectors of the economy have. After an initial flurry of start-ups, the pace of health-related Internet initial public offerings (IPOS) has slowed. In 1999, 18 e-health companies completed IPOS or secondary stock offerings, raising over $1.2 billion in capital, according to investment banking firm Bear Stearns & Company (Halter 2000). In the third quarter of 1999, nearly 16 percent ($153 million) of the total investments directed at healthcare companies went to Internet ventures, up from only 3 percent in the second quarter. Bear Stearns' investment analysts predict that $70 billion in medical products may be moving through e-commerce channels within five years, and e-health companies' revenues will grow to $17.5 billion in the United States, totaling $35 billion worldwide. Healthcare's $1.3 trillion annual expenditures are the target for Internet entrepreneurs seeking to turn the health industry's billions of transactions into billions in revenues.

Venture capital is still flowing to Internet companies. Through the third quarter of 2000, some $40 billion of venture capital was placed with Internet-specific offerings, whereas only $2.7 billion went to medical- and health-related concerns (Smith 2000). This continued infusion sustains optimism for the future of e-health and indicates new market channels for potential healthcare partners. Primary targets for B2B Web-enabled solutions in healthcare include:

- supply-chain management;
- electronic claims and billing;
- acceleration of revenues;
- business process improvement;
- human resources processes;
- managed care processes; and
- health insurance marketing and sales.

In this new millennium, healthcare providers have two reasons to apply e-health strategies—increasing top-line revenues and reducing expenses. E-health initiatives are relatively inexpensive. Much of the infrastructure already exists in computer networks and legacy IT systems. Communications costs are falling rapidly, and Internet access is virtually universal among healthcare providers. The combination of e-health initiatives like "e-cash" and online auction purchasing can be applied directly to the bottom line at a time when many providers' finances have been hit hard by the Balanced Budget Act and the downturn in the stock market, which has reduced investment income.

WILL THE INTERNET REINVENT HEALTHCARE?

Every healthcare CEO is asking how the Internet will affect their business. The answer is that the Internet gives healthcare managers an industrial-strength tool kit to reengineer and improve the delivery system, as well as to streamline back-office functions like human resources and supply-chain management (Hochstadt and Lewis 1999). The Internet is a low-cost, continuously accessible mechanism for bringing people and information together on a 24×7 basis without regard for distance or time zones.

Watching from the sidelines is not an option: In the new economy, healthcare organizations must aggressively explore and exploit Internet opportunities. Organizations that do not want to participate in Internet commerce may be forced to do so by competitors or customers (Ghosh 1998).

The digital transformation scenario for healthcare has moved more slowly in part due to a capital shortage. The financial impact of the BBA has been devastating to IT capital budgets and IS upgrades. Since 1997, the BBA has cut nearly $200 billion in Medicare payments, sharply reducing capital spending plans in every U.S. hospital and health system. Budgets for information technology were slashed by one-third in the year 2000 but should improve in 2001–2005. Predictions by chief information officers in the annual Leadership Survey by HIMSS foresee an upturn in capital spending and new systems installations, now that Congress has provided hospitals with more than $11 billion in BBA reimbursement relief for 2000 (HIMSS 2001).

Since Y2K, tight budgets have forced legacy information systems and software vendors to better demonstrate their "value proposition" and "business case" to healthcare CIOS and CEOS. Legacy systems have been struggling in a difficult selling environment; hospitals and health systems have deferred many IT investments following the necessary

Table 4.2: Potential Savings to U.S. Healthcare Systems from E-Healthcare B2B Transactions

E-Healthcare Benefit	Potential Savings ($ in Billions)
Efficient product movement	$ 6.7
Efficient information storage	2.6
Efficient order management	1.7
Total	$11.0

Source: U.S. Bancorp Piper Jaffray, cited in Halter (2000, p. 119).

upgrades to achieve Y2K compliance. New financial models are being introduced that respond to hospitals' constrained budget situation. Companies with the staff and infrastructure to provide outsourced healthcare IT services are emerging with new business models as application service providers (ASPS) and business service providers (BSPS). New pricing models on a per-click, per-transaction, per-bed, or monthly subscription basis offer alternatives for hospitals and health systems seeking to reduce their total cost of ownership and share new technology in arrangements that resemble earlier models of time-shared remote data processing systems. Investment in B2B applications could more than offset the upfront costs to providers. Potential savings to the U.S. healthcare system from e-commerce could total $11 billion, according to estimates by U.S. Bancorp Piper Jaffray (see Table 4.2).

Another barrier to e-commerce in healthcare has been the lack of standards for electronic transactions. This hurdle should finally be overcome within two years, when federal regulations for HIPAA are fully implemented by 2003. The new standards will guarantee universal electronic communications connectivity for e-commerce, with complete data confidentiality and patient privacy. Voluntary efforts are also underway to facilitate e-commerce: Group purchasing organizations (GPOS) representing more than two-thirds of U.S. hospitals have partnered with three healthcare B2B exchanges. Their goal is to push manufacturers and distributors of medical supplies to adopt standard product codes simplifying the buying of healthcare products online (Hensley 2000). The buyer consortium, calling itself the "e-standards work group," hopes to compel medical supply makers to adopt universal product numbers and bar codes.

Healthcare has been lagging behind the information revolution. Other businesses are being rapidly reinvented on the Net: Stock brokers and travel agents are being disintermediated by Internet companies that make buying stock or airline tickets at the best prices a fast, cheap process. Customer service and information is available online, will health insurance be next? Internet companies such as HealthAxis .com and healthinsurance.com are expecting small businesses and the self-insured to shop online for customized, low-cost health insurance products. Benefits consultants, including Hewitt, Mercer, Wyatt, and Towers Perrin are developing new options for Fortune 500 self-insured companies, which may switch from defined benefits to e-enabled defined contribution strategies.

Traditional health plans may be disintermediated, unless they reinvent themselves online and prepare to compete with low-cost, high-speed Internet competitors. The potential market of 160 million employer-sponsored employees, dependents, and retirees armed with vouchers or employer contributions will choose from an Internet menu of health plan choices. Hewitt has already announced the formation of a new division, Sageo, the initial market strategy of which focuses on pre-Medicare retirees. Aetna, Cigna, and a number of Blue Cross plans are rapidly launching Internet initiatives of their own.

One reason healthcare has lagged behind the Internet revolution has been physician resistance. But that is changing rapidly, as doctors in increasing numbers join the universe of Internet users at home, in the medical office, and in the hospital. The Internet promises to make doctors more efficient, increasing their revenues, lowering their operating costs, and promoting quality outcomes. Within the next three to five years, physician reliance on the Internet and information technology will be universal. The mouse and the wireless PDA, which can take and transmit dictation, will reinvent the daily practice of medicine (Hochstadt and Lewis 1999, p. 4).

IBN MAY REPLACE IDN

The World Wide Web is redefining IDN—integrated delivery network—as IBN—integrated business network. Pick your integration strategy: horizontal, vertical, or virtual. All healthcare integration strategies can now be migrated to the Web. The Internet provides the "glue" for low-cost and seamless integration; Internet-enabled connectivity will be facilitated by higher-speed telecommunications networks. Communications companies are rushing to connect the world with fiber-optic, cable, satellite-based, and wireless networks. Data compression technologies are dramatically expanding the capability and transmission speed of all media, including America's most familiar communications networks—the twin copper wires of the telephone companies. Wireless PDAS like the Palm Pilot and Microsoft's Pocket PC are providing the models for the medical records of the future, which will be handheld, wireless, and capable of recording and transmitting voice as well as data. Data warehouses will provide secure, confidential data storage and retrieval for doctors, hospitals, benefits managers, and health plans. Ultimately consumers will have the ability to create and maintain personal electronic medical records (PEMRS).

The Internet is the next battleground for control of the health industry. A number of competing IBN sponsors include healthcare organizations, HMOS and PPOS, GPOS, physician practice management (PPM) companies, and Internet entrepreneurs like WebMD. Making the transition to the information economy requires a health organization with the vision and financial leverage to combine a hospital system with physician office systems into an integrated business network (Gross 2000). In addition, providers must pick up the pace of implementing e-health strategies.

B2B EXCHANGES

Online B2B exchanges are rapidly changing how business purchases everything from raw materials to highly finished technology. Across American commerce, exchanges are challenging traditional buyer-distributor-seller relationships. Over 100 industry sectors now have B2B firms that offer lowest-cost pricing with rapid shipping and quality guarantees (Sculley and Woods 1999). The concept of "premium pricing" even for new products is being challenged by B2B exchanges, which are converting a huge array of traditional products, and even services, into commodities. In the new economy, few traditional suppliers, even the pharmaceutical giants Merck and Johnson & Johnson, can refuse to do business with B2B exchanges.

In healthcare, new B2B start-ups like Neoforma and medibuy are moving rapidly into strategic business alliances and mergers with the largest group purchasing organizations. A series of Internet business alliances are rapidly being formed, linking e-commerce companies with giant healthcare GPOs like VHA of Irving, Texas, and California-based American Healthcare Systems in La Jolla. Together, they are creating new joint-venture companies like VHA and Neoforma's Novation to serve their old-line customer base with online pricing and cost savings. Medibuy recently purchased Premier Health Exchange, the e-commerce company launched by Premier, the second-largest buyer of hospital supplies, and medibuy made a similar deal with HCA–The Healthcare Company, acquiring HCA's e-commerce business, empact-Health.com (*Modern Healthcare Daily* 2001). Traditional old economy businesses such as sales of used medical equipment to third-world countries have been transformed into a new economy online global auction for medical equipment, supplies, and products.

E-HEALTH STRATEGIES FOR BOOSTING REVENUES, CUTTING COSTS

The Internet will efficiently connect the disparate parties within healthcare and enable universal, affordable access and management of information. Web-based technology offers a practical solution for transforming the fragmented, inefficient healthcare industry from its dependence on "bits of paper to bytes of data" (Hochstadt and Lewis 1999). In the information era, healthcare executives need to recognize the new fundamentals for doing business successfully:

- Healthcare is a transactions business, and the Internet is the lowest-cost venue for electronic commerce.
- Healthcare has significantly underinvested in information technology and has limited in-house expertise.
- Providers must have continuous, instantaneous connectivity with physicians, health plans, and suppliers.
- Cost and revenue breakthroughs will be achieved when routine transactions occur system to system.
- Many existing clinical and business functions can be automated and migrated to the Web.
- First movers will gain significant strategic advantages over slower-to-adapt competitors.

In the next five years, the electronic health market will invest in a number of B2B strategies with significant revenue and cost effects.

Physician Transactions

Medical offices are well behind hospitals in applications of e-commerce. Barely 40 percent of physician claims to insurers are submitted electronically, compared with 95 to 98 of percent electronic claims by hospitals. Many routine medical office functions are performed manually, including patient scheduling, day-before appointment reminders, verification of insurance eligibility, prior treatment authorization by payers, patient visit and progress notes, laboratory data, referrals to other sources of care, and medical office claims to payers. Doctors anecdotally report they routinely spend two to three hours each day on paperwork and telephone time with insurance companies. As much as 60 to 70 percent of physician office staff time and overhead expenses are devoted to maintenance of paper records and manual systems.

The Internet has the potential to reinvent both the business of medicine and the practice of medicine. Physician use of the Internet is rising rapidly, doubling in the past two years. According to the American Medical Association, 37 percent of physicians now use the Internet in

Figure 4.1: Growth in U.S. Physicians' Use of the World Wide Web, 1997–99

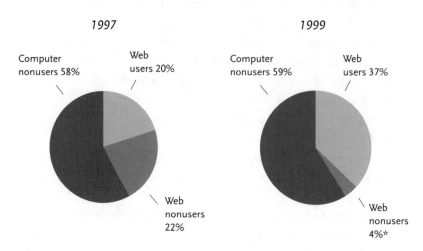

*In 1999, 58 percent of these physicians said they planned to acquire Internet access in the next six months.

Source: American Medical Association, "2000 AMA Study on Physicians' Use of the World Wide Web," cited in Halter (2000, p. 119).

their offices (see Figure 4.1), most on a daily basis (Halter 2000). Current Web use by physicians is more often related to obtaining information for medical, administrative, and insurance purposes, but clinical use of the Internet is growing. Hospital-employed physicians are migrating to the Web at a much faster rate. According to a national survey by VHA, use of the Internet by physicians employed by VHA-member hospitals jumped from 28 percent in 1998 to 82 percent in 1999 (Stevens 2000). Companies like Healtheon/WebMD are investing heavily to improve physician Internet connectivity and to promote Internet-based transactions inside and outside the physician office.

Doctors are learning that medicine is a transaction business. An analysis of a typical patient visit to a physician's office includes 12 common transactions, including (Hochstadt and Lewis 1999):

1. scheduling an appointment;
2. registering of patient-and payer-specific information;
3. verifying coverage and benefit eligibility;
4. ordering treatment of diagnostic testing;
5. requesting follow-up care, for example, follow-up visits, referral care;
6. requesting payer prior authorization;
7. writing and filling prescriptions;
8. reviewing payer (and pharmacy benefit management company) formularies for coverage of prescription orders;
9. receiving test results and communicating them to patients;
10. submitting clinical documentation to payers;
11. generating bills for patients and payers; and
12. coding services provided and submitting claims to third-party payers.

Processing today's healthcare transactions is a labor-intensive process that is slow, time consuming, costly, and sometimes inaccurate. Today, these transactions are processed using the telephone, fax, and mail, with the provider bearing the major cost burden of preparing information. Worse yet, the current system offers payers many excuses to deny claims or return them as incomplete. The delay gives payers the opportunity to arbitrage the "float" of investment income from unpaid claims, while providers fume in endless waits for payment. Doctors in New York, Texas, and other states are filing lawsuits to accelerate payments from HMOs, but they are missing the real point. If every physician office was automated, computer-to-computer electronic claims could be verified and paid in a mouse click.

Managed Care Processes

HMOs and health plans are spending hundreds of millions of dollars on information technology to improve the efficiency of their administrative processes. The collapse of the Oxford Health Plans computer system in 1997–98 only reinforced the proposition that scaling up IT systems was a competitive imperative for successful managed care companies. United, Aetna US Healthcare, and a number of Blue Cross plans have invested heavily in new information technology to manage their costs of doing business. Healtheon's strong move to become a major new player in the electronic data interchange business is a threat to established managed care plans. Some of the nation's leading health insurers, including Aetna, CIGNA, Wellpoint Health Networks, Oxford Health Plans, Foundation Health Systems, and PacifiCare Health, recently announced a strategic partnership to create a joint network for medical claims and managed care transactions to be directly processed over the Internet (Halter 2000).

Managed care organizations are focusing on automation of referral, authorization, claims, eligibility, and reporting (RACER) functions (Hochstadt and Lewis 1999). The survey by AHA identifying the top ten most wired among a sample of HMOS and health plans across the United States (Solovy 2000a) found that four Blue Cross–Blue Shield plans won the most-wired designation, as did two provider-sponsored health plans in Gallup, New Mexico, and Rockford, Illinois. Aggregate data for the most versus least-wired plans showed significant differences in the level of Internet-enabled managed care processes such as member services, consumer health information, disease management, employee and employer services, agent and broker services, and online linkages with providers and suppliers.

B2B Exchanges

One of the most promising Internet business models is the B2B exchange, creating online markets that unite buyers and sellers (Sculley and Woods 1999). Improving the efficiency of purchasing and product movement could yield $8.4 billion in Internet-enabled savings (see Table 4.3), more than two-thirds of the $11 billion potential savings from e-healthcare B2B transactions, according to estimates by U.S. Bancorp Piper Jaffray (Halter 2000). The healthcare industry spends more than $100 billion annually in the United States on medical products and services (Meyer 2000a). As mentioned earlier, Internet start-ups like Neoforma and medibuy.com are hoping to provide a "better,

Table 4.3: Comparing Most-Wired and Least-Wired Hospitals, 2000

Online Application/Process	Most Wired (%)	Least Wired (%)
Appointment scheduling	10.0	2.2
Physician referral	66.0	27.5
Access patient data	58.0	13.2
Clinical pathways	35.0	8.8
Lab order entry	29.0	14.4
Pathology order entry	29.0	3.3
Pharmacy order entry	25.0	2.2
Case management	11.0	1.1
Claims submission	16.0	3.3
Electronic funds transfer	7.0	0.0
Eligibility verification	33.0	11.0
Precertification	22.0	7.7
Referral authorization	19.0	3.3
Medical-surgical suppliers online (81–100%)	25.0	5.1
Pharmacy suppliers online (81–100%)	36.8	12.4

Source: Solovy (2000a, p. 35).

faster, cheaper" alternative to GPOs and traditional buyer-distributor-seller relationships. Neoforma announced a joint venture in March 2001 with Eclipsys Corp and HEALTHvision Inc. to create a new B2B marketplace serving e-healthcare.

In reaction to what may be perceived by suppliers in the industry as the Internet threat, a number of the nation's largest healthcare suppliers announced in late March 2001 they were jointly forming an online exchange that will use the Internet to link provider purchasers with giant supply companies like Johnson & Johnson, GE Medical Systems, Baxter International, Abbott Laboratories, and Medtronic (Meyer 2000b). Customers will not pay transaction fees, as with other online exchanges. Hospital purchasing agents will negotiate contracts with suppliers, as they do now, but will make all their purchases through the suppliers' B2B exchange. Providers can make repeated buys at preset prices with only a keyboard stroke, eliminating the hassles of faxes and phone calls to participating suppliers. Other vendors are joining the alliance, including Boston Scientific, Becton Dickinson, and Guidant Corp. Companies like GE Medical Systems are anticipating that they can boost annual revenues by $50 to $100 million, even if they have to sacrifice traditional pricing to win online business.

Electronic Shopping Carts

Online medical buying (OLMB) applications are evolving as one of the fastest-growing sectors of B2B (Vogel 2000b). The goal is to migrate most of the $150 billion market for medical supplies, equipment, and pharmaceuticals to the Web, as well as the $800 million market for used medical equipment. More than 98 percent of all hospital supplies are purchased using a mix of traditional paper-based, highly manual systems with automated inventory-based electronic purchasing. Electronic order entry systems are widely installed in U.S. hospitals, linking providers with GPOs and suppliers. This e-commerce technology is well suited for high-volume, repetitive daily purchases, which constitute about 50 percent of all medical-surgical supplies and 80 percent of drugs (Halter 2000). Bar-coded medical, surgical, and pharmaceutical products are maintained on a continuous electronic inventory and reordered automatically as the order entry system sends notification that products are being consumed.

This relatively inflexible hospital-centric system is now being reinvented by the Internet. Four Internet companies are competing for market position in OLMB, including Neoforma.com, Cimtek Commerce, medibuy.com, and MedSite, and are developing strategic business relationships with GPOs. Across the continuum of care, physician offices, long-term-care facilities, and many other provider settings can now be connected by low-cost Internet systems to obtain the purchasing power and savings of automated ordering and supply-chain management. Neoforma in particular is an innovator in healthcare B2B. The company has focused on content accuracy and completeness in its electronic presentation of medical equipment and supplies. Purchasers can view Neoforma products in a "virtual hospital," which provides displays of more than 1,000 examination and special procedure rooms, manipulating images that rotate 360 degrees. Cimtek's medicalbuyer .com offers a catalog of products aggregated from wholesalers, not directly from manufacturers. Purchasers receive information directly from the wholesale community, which is traditionally less expensive than purchasing direct (Vogel 2000b).

The expanded healthcare e-commerce market is causing many suppliers and GPOs to rethink their business strategies. Doing business on the Web requires transactions to be transparent to buyers and sellers. Assuming that e-commerce in healthcare follows a pattern similar to direct-to-consumer Internet buying, healthcare suppliers will have to reveal their prices to potential customers—and the competition. Large buyers like GPOs could see their discounts revealed to the marketplace, which could level the playing field between smaller and larger suppliers and among customers. Reverse auctioning will put Internet-based suppliers on equal footing, competing on price until the lowest price to the buyer emerges.

Purchaser Internet Buying Alliances

Traditional GPOs are scrambling to reinvent themselves for Internet competition. GPOs like Premier and VHA-sponsored Novation have driven the price of many healthcare products and pharmaceuticals down to commodity levels but are frustrated that many of their hospital and health system members buy only 50 percent of their supplies through the GPOs. The $200 billion market of medical supplies and products is ripe for Internet-based purchasing organizations. Analysts estimate that 15 to 35 percent of supplies and pharmaceuticals could be bought and sold on the Internet, a potential $30 to $70 billion revenue market for healthcare B2B companies (Halter 2000). GPOs fear that Internet-based B2B exchanges could disintermediate the role of the GPO in the buyer-seller relationship for health products and medical supplies. The fears are real. Hospitals and health systems are discovering Internet competitors, which deal direct and online, offering lower prices and supply-chain management infrastructure without any initial investment expense, unlike the GPOs, whose members must pay fees to join the purchasing organizations.

For-profit hospital management companies have been quick to realize the potential of the Internet to reduce their supply costs. Tenet Healthcare Corporation has formed an Internet purchasing alliance, Broadlane, in a joint venture with Ventro Corporation. More than 250 hospitals will combine their online buying power through Broadlane, including 113 hospitals in the Santa Barbara, California–based Tenet health system (Meyer 2000b). Columbia/HCA (now HCA Healthcare), the nation's largest for-profit hospital chain, is investing up to $40 million in empactHealth.com, a B2B e-healthcare company that offers automated catalog ordering of medical-surgical supplies and is moving into Web-based purchasing from online portal-to-portal vendor inventories. HCA's 200 member hospitals spend $3 billion annually on health and medical supplies.

The convergence of GPOs and Internet exchanges is a rapidly emerging trend, with the largest group purchasing organizations solidifying Internet alliances in the past few months. Premier, the largest healthcare GPO serving nonprofit hospitals and health systems, recently announced it would partner with medibuy.com (Halter 2000). Under the agreement, San Diego–based Premier's Internet subsidiary, Premier Health Exchange, has been sold to medibuy. Premier CEO Rick Norling announced that the deal would give Premier a more comprehensive approach in the rapidly growing B2B exchange business than the GPO could have achieved on its own. Premier will gain seats on medibuy's board, as well as a six-year exclusive contract as Premier's e-commerce infrastructure supplier. Medibuy is free to sell to other GPOs, provider organizations, and health plans.

The healthcare B2B exchange market is rapidly shaping into a battle of two giants—medibuy and Neoforma. VHA, the second-largest GPO, based in Irving, Texas, quickly responded to Premier's medibuy alliance by announcing an exclusive ten-year deal with Neoforma. The Neoforma relationship will be managed through Novation, a joint venture chiefly funded by VHA and the University HealthSystem Consortium (UHC), which will channel the purchasing power of 6,500 healthcare organizations through Novation and Neoforma. The deal with

Novation goes hand in hand with the $1.45 billion acquisition by Neo-forma of Eclipsys, a healthcare software and services company, and its affiliate HEALTHvision. VHA and UHC will receive a combined 30 percent in the resulting e-commerce company. To illustrate the immensity of the deal, Neoforma has assembled a database of 400,000 health and medical supply items from 15,000 vendors.

Online Pharmacies

Internet-minded firms are accelerating the transition of pharmacy to the Web. Emerging in 1999, online pharmacies such as PlanetRx, drugstore.com, cranespharmacy.com, and cvs.com have been competing for mind share and market share, but with limited success so far. Online drug stores are still struggling to achieve significant revenues, and profits are still far in the future. Market-entry hurdles like 50-state licensing have been time consuming, and national health plans have been slow to recognize the online pharmacies as authorized sources of prescription drugs for their enrollees. The online market for prescription drugs and other drugstore products has no clear leader yet, and traditional pharmacy chains like cvs are entering the competition. Seeking to raise their visibility with consumers, some online pharmacy companies are partnering with other Internet e-tailing companies, like Amazon.com, which has acquired a 40 percent share of drugstore .com.

Compelling doctors to write drug prescriptions online is far from universal, even after enactment of federal legislation authorizing the use of electronic signatures in 2000. A number of barriers remain before widespread physician acceptance of online prescribing is achieved. According to a recent report in *Drug Store News,* less than one percent of U.S. physicians are currently writing electronic prescriptions (Halter 2000). Companies targeting the e-prescription market include eScript, LogonHealth, Advanced Health Technologies, iScribe, ePhysician, Proxymed, and Allscripts. Companies already offering e-prescribing include Healtheon/WebMD, PlanetRx.com, and eMD.com. Currently only a limited number of drugstores are electronically enabled, but the large drugstore chains are evaluating the technology now and should have the infrastructure in place for e-prescribing by 2002.

As a result, pure Internet companies may be cannibalized by drug wholesalers or health plans. Pharmaceutical wholesalers like Bergen Brunswick, McKesson/HBOC, and Cardinal Health are building or buying online pharmacy businesses. Wholesalers may outcompete the Internet start-ups with their long-standing relationships with pharmaceutical manufacturers, relations with pharmacy benefit management companies, and experience in handling all types of pharmaceuticals, including narcotics (Vogel 2000b). Most importantly, drug wholesalers have the volume to get the best prices from pharmaceutical manufacturers, while Internet start-ups will not have the established volume to get the same level of discounts from the drug makers. This year, McKesson launched Internet services for independent drugstores, allowing pharmacists to create their own web sites at which customers can order prescription refills and obtain information about pharmaceuticals (Meyer 2000a). Drug distributor Cardinal unveiled Chain-Online in December 1999, which also creates customized web sites for chain pharmacies. Although slow at the outset and facing significant barriers, pharmacies are rapidly joining the information age. Some 87 percent of all pharmacies have web sites, according to the National Association of Chain Drug Stores.

Despite aggressive predictions for volume and revenue growth, online pharmacies are still struggling to capture a significant piece of the $160 billion annual drug expenditures. Many consumers still cannot buy pharmaceuticals online because their HMO will not reimburse them. Drugstore.com and PlanetRx.com report they are turning away 90 percent of consumer inquiries because the enrollees' health plans do not yet allow patients to purchase drugs at Internet sites using their standard copayments (Stevens 2000). Thus far, no HMOs have their own online drugstores, but many health plans may be offering their online drug refills and consumer information to their enrollees by 2002. Internet pharmacy companies are partnering with pharmacy benefit management (PBM) companies to gain access to the PBMS' mail-order pharmacy relationships with the health plans, but this is not exactly e-tailing. For example, online pharmacies are partnering with national drug chains like Rite Aid and cvs to gain market share and distribution networks. PlanetRx has recently announced an innovative partnership with Helios Health, which is installing an "e-station" Internet connection in doctors' waiting rooms. Consumers can ask health questions through the e-station, respond to special offers, and order prescriptions after their doctor's examination.

Disease Management

Disease management is a prime target for Internet applications, but migrating care coordination to the Web is taking longer than anticipated. In a surprising survey result from aha, most-wired hospitals offer more consumer health information than health plans about 11 highly prevalent disease conditions such as asthma, depression, stroke, and hiv (Solovy 2000a). Few hospitals or health plans take disease management much further into cyberspace. Only a small number of plans or hospitals provide online nurse triage or Internet-based health risk assessments; nor do they offer the ability for patients to report self-administered test results such as diabetic sugar levels.

Internet-enabled disease management is targeting high-risk, chronically ill patient populations like those suffering from hypertension, heart disease, asthma, and diabetes. The fda has recently approved a heart monitoring device, the Tracker, owned by Tiarong Building Materials Holdings of New York (Halter 2000). This battery-powered device provides ekg signals via a continuous-loop, digital memory recorder, which can be worn up to 30 days. Event data are transmitted to remote computers for monitoring and analysis and for building a personal database. Another heart monitoring device offered by Micromedical Industries of Australia achieved worldwide attention in June 1999, when marathoner Pat Farmer telemonitored his heartbeat during a 90-minute run in a live Internet broadcast.

Web Site Development and Hosting

As the number of hospital-sponsored web sites grows, one electronic business emerging is the development and hosting of health-related web sites for consumers or e-commerce. HealthCentral.com, a leading provider of health content and e-commerce services, recently spun off Windom Health Enterprises, which will specialize in web sites for integrated delivery networks, hospitals, and physician group practices. HealthCentral clients include Scripps Clinic in La Jolla, California, Catholic Healthcare West (CHW), and San Francisco–based Brown and Toland medical group, whose independent physician association affiliates 1,600 doctors in Northern California. Interestingly, CHW's web site won three awards at the 1999 eHealthcareWorld Conference in New York.

THE DIGITAL DIVIDE AMONG HEALTHCARE PROVIDERS

A digital divide is emerging among the nation's 5,000 community hospitals. A recent survey by the American Hospital Association found significant differences in Internet savvy and business applications (Solovy 2000a). The top 100 most-wired hospitals submitted an average of 16 percent of their health claims electronically, versus the least-wired facilities, which averaged 3 percent of online claims submissions. The survey indicated clearly that most hospitals fell into the least-wired category. Other significant differences emerge when comparing online precertifications, referral authorizations, and clinical applications such as laboratory, pharmacy, and radiology order entry (see Table 4.3).

LOOKING FORWARD: SURFING THE INTERNET WAVE WITHOUT FALLING OFF

Business immaturity, lack of processes, few trusted business partners, and lack of standard business guidelines will prevent many potentially cost-saving e-businesses from coming to fruition. Online firms must proceed under current acceptable business practices; those waiting for Internet-oriented regulations to evolve will miss early market adoption (Vogel 2000a, p. 1). Migrating many of healthcare's business processes to the Internet offers great promise. Better business solutions, lower prices, and customized processes and products are all possible.

But read the prospectus for healthcare e-commerce carefully. Doing business on the Web may be risky, and providers may find themselves in e-limbo without a safety net. Online medical buying could save 15 to 20 percent with lowest-cost transaction costs, product standardization, adherence to contract compliance, and enterprise best practices (Vogel 2000a). The savings are very attractive to financially strapped healthcare providers, but some arrangements involve new companies and untested processes. Even where the partners in joint-venture B2B exchanges are well known, their online capabilities to cooperate and deliver are still to be proven.

As hundreds of digital electronic marketplaces continue to roll out at Internet speed, e-commerce experts predict that only two to three Internet companies will survive and become profitable in each industry before burning through their venture capital (Long 2000). The battle for control of e-commerce in healthcare is already forcing rapid consolidation, and the e-newcomers are forming strategic relationships with traditional wholesalers, group purchasing organizations, and distributors. Healthcare is traditionally slow to adopt new technologies and management innovations. Hospital and health system CEOs are understandably skeptical about investing in e-health strategies after witnessing the meltdown of the dot-com companies in late 1999 and early 2000.

Even the most successful Internet companies with millions of customers and millions in revenues have struggled to gain profitability, and some have recently failed. Price-earnings ratios are exceedingly high for many publicly traded firms in this sector, and stock values are depressed. In addition, not all of the healthcare Internet start-ups know much about healthcare. Alden Solovy advises that the best dot-coms will be those that find the magic combination of old-economy healthcare expertise and new-economy tech savvy, with a mix of technical skills and health-organization expertise in senior management (Solovy 2000b).

Not every Internet commerce venture will survive. Hembrech & Quist recently gave a negative assessment for the prospects of the New Health Exchange, a Web-based B2B exchange jointly funded by AmeriSource Health Corporation, Cardinal Health, Fisher Scientific,

McKesson/HBOC, and Owens & Minor. H&Q's analysts fear that the suppliers' grand aspirations will face an enormous technologic task, and the venture needs to answer many questions before it proceeds (Meyer 2000a). The idea of multifirm "co-opetition"—a combination of competition and cooperation—is very attractive, and the sponsoring firms have excellent industry reputations, but the partnership must demonstrate that online collaboration will yield both low price and value-added service.

But it's early in the Internet revolution. The first cycle of boom and bust on the Internet is being replaced by a longer, stronger up-cycle of larger, better-capitalized firms with solid business plans and experienced management. Consolidation is occurring between traditional legacy healthcare information technology vendors and "born on the Web" companies, and lines are blurring between old and new competitors. Internet-based B2B newcomers are finding that elbowing their way into long-standing relationships between buyers and suppliers is not easy (Hamel 2000). Long-established vendors like Johnson & Johnson and Baxter are fighting back by starting their own B2B exchanges. J&J has been joined by GE Medical Systems, Baxter International, Abbott Laboratories, and Medtronic, investing hundreds of millions of dollars and vowing to match price cuts and resist disintermediation by Internet start-ups. The five companies currently manufacture about 70 percent of the supplies, equipment, and drugs bought by the nation's hospitals (Halter 2000).

B2B winners and losers will be sorted out in the next 12 to 18 months. Lower price is obviously the driving factor in the Internet migration for purchasers, but price is not the ultimate differentiator among competing e-health firms. The keys to success are to offer end-to-end solutions for customers, provide software that services the entire process, have the capability to scale up as the business grows, and provide value-added services. Internet business guru Dr. Ravi Kalokota, author of *e-Business: Roadmap for Success,* advises companies moving their business processes to the Web that customer care may be the ultimate decision factor after e-businesses have driven down prices to their lowest levels (Long 2000). Next-generation B2B players will partner with existing distributors in a clicks-and-bricks strategy to assure immediate and complete fulfillment of customer orders and provide value-added services such as customized data and reports (Gray Sheet 2000). At the end of the day, buyer-seller relationships are still concerned with quality, service, and value, even in the new economy.

STRATEGIC IMPLICATIONS

Ignore the hype about the Internet, and make plans to participate in B2B cost-effective solutions across a wide range of business transactions.

Do Not Underestimate the Internet. It would be a mistake to overreact to the Wall Street collapse of many of the dot-com companies. Moving business to the Internet is a long-term trend for every sector of the economy. Follow progress closely in other sectors; they can illustrate productive opportunities for healthcare organizations, for example, supply-chain management, advancing receivables, and disintermediating all those third parties in transaction processes that do not add value.

Evaluate B2B Opportunities. Utilize outside consultants to evaluate the range of B2B business opportunities. Do not assume that mid-level managers are capable of assessing B2B potential in their arenas. More likely, some managers will see the Internet as a threat, not an opportunity.

Invest in the Future. Not every organization is ready or able to be an early adopter, but everyone can be an early observer. Invest in making business functions Internet ready and initiate Internet solutions with frequent evaluation. Be patient for results. They may not arise with Internet speed, but the genie is out of the bottle on this trend. B2B will be the way of things to come.

REFERENCES

Carrns, A. 2001. "Dot.Com Rx: Veteran Entrepreneur Treats Ailing WebMD with Strong Medicine." *Wall Street Journal,* January 17, pp. A1, A19.

Coile, R. C., Jr. 2000. "'B2B' Healthcare Strategies Harness the Internet for Business." *Health Trends* 12 (10): 1–12.

———. 2001. *Futurescan 2001: A Millennium Forecast of Healthcare Trends 2001–2005*, p. 1–32. Chicago: Health Administration Press and American Hospital Association.

Evans, P., and T. S. Wurster. 2000. *Blown to Bits: How the New Economics of Information Transforms Strategy.* Boston: Harvard Business School Press.

Ghosh, S. 1998. "Making Business Sense of the Internet." *Harvard Business Review* 76 (2): 126–35.

Gray Sheet. 2000. "Clicks and Bricks Both Needed for Success of Device B2B E-Commerce," pp. 1–3. Chevy Chase, MD: F-D-C Reports, Inc.

Gross, W. D. 2000. Personal correspondence. Medimetrix Consulting, Cleveland, OH, May 24.

Halter, P. 2000. "The E-Health Revolution." *MedPro Month* 10 (4): 1, 118–25.

Hamel, G. 2000. "Will the 'Frictionless Economy' Slip You Up?" *Wall Street Journal,* June 6, p. A26.

Hensley, S. 2000. "Hospital Co-Ops Seek to Ease Purchases on Web." *Wall Street Journal,* June 14, p. B2.

Healthcare Information Management Systems Society (HIMSS). 2001. "12th Annual HIMSS Leadership Survey." Preliminary results, pp. 1–28. Chicago: HIMSS.

Hochstadt, B., and D. Lewis. 1999. Bits of Paper to Bytes of Data: A White Paper on Healthcare and the Internet. San Francisco: Thomas Weisel Partners.

Lewis, M. 2000. *The New New Thing: A Silicon Valley Story.* New York: W. W. Norton and Co.

Long, S. 2000. "E-Commerce Pioneer Predicts Winners of B2B e-Marketplace Consolidation." *PR Newswire,* May 31, pp. 1–5.

Meyer, C. 2000a. "E-Marketplace Will Help Cut Costs, Set Industry Standards, Healthcare Distributors Say." [Online news report.] Skila, Inc. April, pp. 1–4. http://www.skila.com.

———. 2000b. "Healthcare Giants Form Online Market." [Online news report.] Skila, Inc., May, pp. 1–4. http://www.skila.com.

Modern Healthcare Daily 2001. "E-Procurement Firm Completes Acquisition." News Tidbits, February 8, p. 2. [Online news brief.] Southfield, MI: Superior Consultant.

Sculley, A. B., and W. A. Woods. 1999. "B2B Exchanges: The Killer Application in the Business-to-Business Internet Revolution." [Online article.] ISI Publications. http://www.isipublications.com.

Solovy, A. 2000a. "Is an E-Commerce Gap Emerging Among the Nation's Hospitals?" *Hospitals & Health Networks* 74 (4): 30–41.

———. 2000b. "The New Economy Would Benefit from Some Old Economy Experience." *Hospitals & Health Networks* 74 (4): 28.

Smith, R. 2000. "Venture Capital Investment Trends." *Wall Street Journal,* December 1, p. C17.

Stevens, L. 2000. "Still Having Growing Pains." *Medicine on the Net* 6 (6): 1–4.

Vogel, D. 2000a. "Online Medical Buying: Part 2—Identifying Differentiation." *Healthcare Information Technology Strategies*, File 226, April 25, pp. 1–2. Stamford, CT: Meta Group.

———. 2000b. "Online Pharmacy: Part 1—Where's the Business?" *Healthcare Information Technology Strategies*, File 224, February 7, pp. 1–2. Stamford, CT: Meta Group.

CHAPTER FIVE

E-Solutions: Harnessing the Internet for Business Improvement

KEY CONCEPTS: *Supply-chain management • E-cash • Hospital-physician intranet • E-transactions • The innovator's dilemma • First-mover advantage*

INTRODUCTION: The digital transformation of healthcare will require hospital organizations, physicians, suppliers, and health plans to adopt Internet connectivity and computer-assisted decision support. The outcome will be to reduce costs, systematically improve clinical quality, and produce optimum patient outcomes. E-solutions will provide new strategies to achieve both cost and revenue goals and will create new relationships with patients, physicians, suppliers, health plans, and government agencies. E-health experts at Superior Consultant project savings in a number of areas, such as:

- supply-chain management strategies;
- e–managed care connections;
- Internet-connected care management programs;
- "e-cash" systems;
- outsourced information systems; and
- intranets for physicians.

"ULTIMATELY, JUST ABOUT everything and everyone will be networked. Internet access will be everywhere, whether from a personal computer, a handheld organizer, a pager, or some other remote communications device. However, being wired does not change human behavior overnight. There will be both technical and cultural challenges while the technology awaits and promotes changes in the way people think and act."

—*Chuck Martin (2000, p. 11)*

Electronic solutions to all aspects of healthcare harness the power of the Internet and information technology in the digital transformation of business processes. On a global level, Internet-based killer applications are being unleashed to transform every industry, economic sector, and business relationship (Downes and Mui 2000, p. 5). Now the Web is going wireless, which should propel the Internet boom forward at an even faster pace. Ignition, a new venture capital firm specializing in wireless Internet companies, raised $140 million and received 100 business plans by the end of its first business day (Schonfeld 2000). According to the recently launched magazine, *e-Company*, there are 214 million wireless customers worldwide; only 24 million of them are in the United States. The global bottom line is simple: faster, cheaper, and better, with low-cost digitization of nearly every device and process.

The business assumptions on which healthcare organizations have been managed are in the process of being replaced by new Internet-based assumptions. The Internet is changing the "way the game is played," with new opportunities for cost savings and revenue enhancement (McCormack 1999). E-health experts at Superior Consultant, an integrated IS and IT consulting firm based in Southfield, Michigan, project savings in a number of areas.

- Supply-chain management strategies give purchasers the lowest-cost access to all products, saving 10 to 15 percent on every purchase.
- E-managed care connections reduce the cost of verifying insurance eligibility from $32 per patient to $0.60; electronic authorization of treatment slashes provider back-office expenses from $16 per case to $1.60.
- Internet-connected care management programs speed laboratory results to physicians, provide computer-based care plans on

Figure 5.1: Growth in Consumers Seeking Health Information on the Web—Harris Poll Data

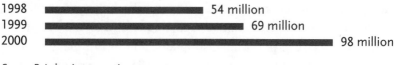

1998 ▆▆▆▆▆▆▆▆▆▆▆▆▆ 54 million
1999 ▆▆▆▆▆▆▆▆▆▆▆▆▆▆▆ 69 million
2000 ▆▆▆▆▆▆▆▆▆▆▆▆▆▆▆▆▆▆▆▆▆ 98 million

Source: Baisden (2000, p. 2).

admission, and lower length of stay by 0.5 to 1.0 days, cutting costs per case by $400 to $1,000 for each patient.

- E-cash systems accelerate electronic claims and payments, reducing days in receivables and pumping millions of dollars into hospital cash flows.
- Outsourcing information systems saves 10 to 15 percent per year, and sale-leaseback of information technology can free up millions of dollars of capital for alternative investments or improved profitability.
- Creation of a hospital or health system intranet for physicians reduces IS and IT operating and capital investment expenses for doctors, and browser-facilitated access to real-time data on their patients enhances physician loyalty, resulting in 10 to 15 percent improvement in physician referrals.

The rapid acceptance by consumers of the Internet as a trusted source for health information is driving healthcare providers, plans, and suppliers to accept and employ the Internet. Healthcare's "e-patients" are becoming savvy browsers of the estimated 15,000 health-related web sites now available on the Internet. The number of people looking to the Web for health information has increased by more than 50 percent in the past two years, to 98 million (see Figure 5.1), according to the latest Harris poll (Baisden 2000). Consumers' experience with Internet shopping indicates that e-patients will expect the same level of choice and responsiveness from healthcare providers and health plans.

DIGITAL TRANSFORMATION MUST DEMONSTRATE RESULTS

Will electronic solutions work in healthcare? For America's $1.3 trillion health industry, the challenge of digital transformation is for healthcare organizations, physicians, suppliers, and health plans to adopt Internet connectivity and computer-assisted decision support to reduce costs, systematically improve clinical quality, and produce optimum patient outcomes. E-solutions will provide new strategies to achieve both cost and revenue goals and create new relationships with patients, physicians, suppliers, health plans, and government agencies.

But are such claims more hype than performance? A growing number of healthcare executives are skeptical about the high cost of ramping up onto the information highway. A recent survey by Gartner Group identified "claims that can't be substantiated" for Internet products and systems as the leading challenge to healthcare information managers (Morrisey 1999). In the months since Y2K, many hospitals and health systems have cut operating IS and IT budgets, deferring capital spending plans for and slowing the pace of upgrading computer systems and software.

CEOs and CIOs are raising concerns about the capital costs, organizational disruption, and lack of positive cost-benefit ratios. High-speed Internet connectivity coupled with enormous expansions of computing power are forcing organizations to change at a dizzying pace. The result for many managers and companies is "blur," in which the pace of change accelerates beyond our comfort zones, according to findings from Ernst & Young's Center for Business Innovation (Davis and Meyer 1998). No longer do clear distinctions exist between structure and process, owning and using, knowing and learning, or real and virtual. The Internet has blurred the boundaries and created new opportunities that take advantage of the Net's superior speed and low-cost connectivity.

A number of barriers remain before providers will switch to e-solutions for many common clinical and business processes. These include the following (Egger 1999):

- *Security concerns.* Although technology exists to guarantee security of patient records, the perception of lack of security is driving the federal government's new HIPAA regulations (Coile 1999).
- *Pace of change.* Growth of the World Wide Web continues at Internet speed, with one million new Web addresses created daily. Healthcare organizations are unaccustomed to this pace of technological change and unwilling to deploy technology that is continually evolving.
- *Physician attitude.* Many doctors continue to be ambivalent toward the information revolution and ease of Internet communications. Physicians who make little use of computers in their offices are reluctant to switch to electronic medical records.
- *Browser limitations.* Browser technologies are simple but can be overwhelmed by the Internet's vast data resources. Complicating the problem of browser limitations, the databases linked by hospital or health system intranets may be loaded with fragmented and out-of-date data.
- *Lack of standards.* Continuing disarray over electronic standards, for example, bar coding, has resulted in many overlapping, competing sets of information in healthcare databases.

Widespread availability of private electronic data interchange systems, such as group purchasing order systems, may also slow the migration of business functions to the Web. Hospitals and group purchasing organizations have millions of dollars of invested capital in private EDI exchanges and may be reluctant to convert to Internet-based systems.

INFORMATION SYSTEMS STILL LAG BEHIND THE NEEDS OF IDNS

As America's 500 integrated health systems and networks grow, they are increasingly dependent on information systems and technology to manage their far-flung facilities and link all IDN-sponsored services into a seamless web of coordinated care. The goal of integrated systems is to build delivery organizations that can capture economies of scale in operations and gain a dominant market share for contracting leverage with managed care organizations.

Ten years of research in the application of information technology in IDNs reveals a mixed case study of progress and frustration. In Stephen Shortell's new book, *Remaking Health Care in America* (Second Edition), Shortell and his coauthors update their decade-long study of integration in leading IDNs across the nation. They report that information systems are a key factor in development of an organized IDN (Shortell et al. 2000). Unfortunately, information systems continue to be a major impediment to integration for all of the case-study IDNs. In spite of the millions of dollars spent by the health systems on IT, all of the IDNs criticized their information systems as inadequate in the critical function of physician and clinical integration. The Shortell team believes that the IDNs have spent most of their IS or IT budget in recent years on Y2K issues and have failed to reach goals such as implementing universal patient identifiers. In the future, improving the reach and functionality of information systems and linking physicians fully will be key factors in IDN development. Shortell and colleagues encourage IDNs to expand the focus of their information systems from business processes to clinical care and quality management.

More than 80 percent of all U.S. hospitals are members or affiliates of integrated systems and networks. The concept of the integrated delivery network is still a work in progress and may even be considered a misnomer (Crozier 2000, p. 8). All too few IDNs are truly integrated from an information standpoint. Inadequate data systems create obvious problems for system-level managers who lack timely data on performance of subunits. In today's environment of declining profits, Medicare budget cuts under the BBA, and proliferation of HMOs, hospitals and health systems face the "information imperative": IDN- or hospitalwide cost cutting requires explicit and timely information. Managed care contracting requires financial and clinical information systems that can identify cost and utilization patterns by payer. Although many providers are withdrawing from capitation and at-risk arrangements, a healthcare organization must still know its costs in fine-grain detail.

For a provider organization to be truly integrated, it must have access to information across its entire business. The Internet makes an ideal data collection and reporting method because it can service a wide geographic area at a low cost (Crozier 2000). Users can access a Web-based system from any location with a land line or cellular telephone service. No additional infrastructure is needed. Despite these advantages, the Internet may not transform healthcare as rapidly as it has revolutionized other industries. Among healthcare's 100 most-wired hospitals and health systems, 100 percent have web sites; among the least wired, so do 97 percent. But connectivity for patients, employees, health plans, and suppliers varies widely and seldom tops 50 percent in any category, even among the most-wired institutions, according to the American Hospital Association's annual survey in *Hospitals & Health Networks* (Solovy 2000). Many legal, regulatory, reimbursement, clinical, and cultural characteristics of healthcare hinder the absorption of technologies, suggests John Glaser, CIO of Boston's Partners HealthCare system (Mjoseth 2000). The construction of the information highway in healthcare is making progress but is still not moving at Internet speed.

E-SOLUTIONS: SEVEN STRATEGIES FOR PERFORMANCE IMPROVEMENT

As the new millennium continues, the Internet will become the "hub of healthcare," predicts John Morrisey, information editor for *Modern Healthcare* (Morrisey 1999). Forget all that you have heard about community health information networks that require your organization to contract with a vendor of proprietary software, supply a copy of that software to every potential user of the network, and support that network with staff. Consider instead what a global open standard network can do for you, your patients, your organization, and your community (Ruffin 1999, p. 73).

The rapid growth of Web-based connectivity is a strong "push" factor for deployment of e-solutions in healthcare. Web-based systems are far easier and less expensive to acquire, maintain, and service than client-server or mainframe-based systems. Many chief information officers believe that the Internet makes provider organizations offers they cannot refuse—lower costs, widespread access, and interface engines for in-place hardware and software. Within this decade, Web technology will eventually replace most traditional models (Kilbridge 2000). Already, the healthcare market is seeing a consolidation of legacy information technology providers with newer intranet companies to offer integrated technology solutions.

Supply-Chain Management

Integrated delivery networks, hospitals of all sizes, and physician group practices are beginning to recognize the value of electronic business strategies in managing workflow and materials across their service areas. Business-to-business activities such as supply-chain management can reduce the costs of supplies and equipment and facilitate other savings using strategies such as just-in-time inventory. In addition to the Internet, more vendors are handling supply transactions by exchanging electronically through either point-to-point computer connections or value-added networks—private networks that store and forward electronic messages. By one estimate, provider organizations could reduce supply costs by $11 billion per year across the nation by using EDI links with supply-chain partners for an array of purchasing activities, such as checking product availability, sending purchase orders, receiving invoices, and processing payments (McCormack 1999, p. 55).

Sophisticated provider organizations have been using private EDI networks for years through national group purchasing organizations such as VHA and Premier. Now the Internet is acting as an equalizer for smaller hospitals and physician groups, with Internet e-commerce vendors giving these smaller buyers similar cost reductions and as-needed delivery services that formerly were only available to the largest purchasers. Larger purchasers may use the Internet for comparison shopping even while they continue to rely primarily on private EDI networks with GPOs or direct electronic interchanges with vendors. Many hospitals buy between 30 and 50 percent of their supplies and equipment outside of their GPOs. A lot of purchasing takes place where the volumes are low, buyers prefer a non-GPO alternative product, or demand is highly variable, for example, from the operating room to the central supply service to the business office.

These purchases could migrate to the Internet, believes Jamie Wyatt, director of healthcare solutions for PeopleSoft, a Pleasanton, California–based software vendor that offers a Web-enabled materials management system (McCormack 1999). An array of new companies is emerging in healthcare's supply-chain management e-commerce space, such as medibuy.com, which offers providers the opportunity to submit requests for proposals to a number of vendors; Medical-Buyer, which offers an Internet buying service, enabling providers to shop for medical products from many different suppliers; and Med-Site.com, which offers a variety of Internet services to medical practices. Allegiance, once a part of Baxter Healthcare, has launched ASAP.e .Comm, a web site that enables providers to order medical and surgical supplies online.

The Internet is providing a new marketplace for buying and selling medical equipment. Neoforma, a Santa Clara, California–based company, provides an online marketplace for buyers and sellers. The availability of an Internet marketplace is a real advantage for large organizations, which in the past often wrote off used equipment because it was difficult to find buyers, as well as for small organizations, which had no effective way to resell their used medical equipment. The Valley Health System, a three-hospital IDN in Hemet, California, is now using Neoforma. William Carik, director of materials management, relates, "People in my position tend to go the path of least resistance and just trade in used equipment to a dealer, even though we know we are not getting the price for it" (McCormack 1999, p. 56).

E-Transactions

A growing number of managed care companies are jumping aboard the Internet and rapidly migrating their enrollee and provider relationships to the Web. Many health plans believe that the low-cost, universally accessible Web will reduce their enrollment costs, link patients with providers, improve customer service, monitor quality, and slash the cost of back-office functions such as eligibility, prior authorization, and physician monitoring. Among the market leaders in the Internet revolution are Aetna US Healthcare, Blue Shield of California, and New York–based Oxford Health Plan.

Internet-based enrollment systems are designed to make signing up for a health plan a quick, low-cost process that can be done directly from an employee's worksite or home computer. Blue Cross of California cut the enrollment cycle from 25 days to 24 hours using online sign-up by brokers through the company's public web site, blueshield-ca.com, with consumers getting almost immediate access to their health benefits (Siwicki 1999). Aetna US Healthcare permits consumers to sign up directly on the "Ezenroll" area of Aetna's web site, using employer-supplied identifications and passwords to employees. In the first six months, Aetna extended Ezenroll to more than 400 employers and 18,000 enrollees and is doubling its plans for Internet-based enrollment.

Automation of medical claims and electronic payments can accelerate payment, lower the average number of days in receivables, and significantly reduce manual labor in the back office. Healthcare providers are increasing efforts to connect with health plans to save money and speed payment. Five of the 100 most-wired hospitals in the United States routinely submit more than 80 percent of their claims online, like Neptune, New Jersey–based Meridian Health Systems. Electronic claims submission tripled last year among the most-wired facilities, but the least wired now submit fewer than one percent of claims (Solovy 2000). The gap between the most- and least-wired hospitals is growing, according to the second annual survey by the American Hospital Association. Hospitals ranked among the best e-connected accomplished 22 percent of precertification online, as well as 33 percent of insurance eligibility checks done electronically. Less-connected hospitals managed barely 10 percent of their managed care transaction over the Internet. Dwayne Jordan, cio of Rehobeth McKinley Christian Hospital in Gallup, New Mexico, predicts, "We expect to move toward handling all transactions online" (Solovy 2000).

Care Management

Many healthcare organizations are using the Internet as a customer channel and communications network, but fewer hospitals and health plans have harnessed the connectivity and distributed computing power of the Internet for day-to-day care management. For years, hospitals beefed up their financial information systems while the automation of medical record keeping lagged. Now the priorities are reversed. Clinical care management is the baseline strategy for helping hospitals regain profitability in the twenty-first century. In Louisiana, the SMA Health Plan manages costs and coordinates care for its 75,000 enrollees utilizing the Clinical Care Viewer, an Internet technology from W3Health, based in Wilmington, Massachusetts (Danaher 2000). This Web browser–based clinical reference system speeds up utilization management reviews by the health plan's care managers with increased productivity, less training, and more time for other value-added tasks such as continuing care management.

To achieve electronic care management capabilities, fundamental improvements are needed in the information infrastructure that supports care management. Nothing less than wholesale process reengineering is required to apply fiscal discipline to clinical costs and to significantly reduce the incidence of medical errors. Dave Garets of the Gartner Group believes that incrementally improving hospitals' existing care processes through total quality management (TQM) will not go far enough or happen fast enough (Mjoseth 2000). A computer-based patient record is the essential building block for clinical reengineering.

Internet-connected care management programs can significantly improve clinical and financial performance. Intranets—electronically connected networks within an organization—can facilitate the presentation of clinical information for doctors and nurses. Data from different legacy systems can now be integrated over intranets for presentation simultaneously on one screen, reducing the need for costly interfaces between once-competing software and hardware (Kilbridge 2000). Web technology, with its platform independence and common user interface, permits clinicians to view data from different systems, such as, laboratory, radiology, or electronic medical records. Some hospitals have begun to provide Web-based browser access to legacy databases. Even for physicians and other caregivers who are not computer literate, the point-and-click simplicity of browser technology can make anyone a Web information user with minimal training.

In Savannah, Georgia, the Memorial Health System has engaged WebMD to link physician offices in a solution that also incorporates access to the Star system, the hospital's clinical database from McKesson/HBOC (Corrales 2000). For $36,000 per year, Memorial received WebMD and Star Clinical Browser connectivity for a core group of 150 physicians. A year later, 447 Memorial physicians are connected to WebMD, and one-third can directly access patient records in the McKesson/HBOC database through the Star Clinical Browser. Although WebMD and McKesson/HBOC now appear to be going in separate directions, Memorial's physicians are gaining confidence in the new system and are asking for two-way Internet communication for placing orders via the Net.

Improving Quality

The 1999 study by the Institute of Medicine on medical errors may ultimately drive enactment of new federal rules for error reporting. Media attention has been critical, and providers have been understandably defensive against charges that 48,000 to 98,000 people may die each year from medical mistakes. The American public believes that a serious problem has been uncovered. Industry observers warn providers that "local Bob Woodwards will be investigating your hospital" (Garets 2000).

Improving quality could save money, maybe lots of it. Quality is a major contributor to success in the annual ratings by HCIA of the top 100 best financially managed hospitals in the United States. Despite the impression that medical errors are widespread, few institutions are using available technology to reduce mistakes. The Institute for Safe Medication Practices estimates that medication errors could be reduced by 85 percent by utilizing simple technologies such as handheld scanners and bar codes, but only 9 percent of U.S. hospitals have purchased handheld technology (Haugh 2000). The Institute also reported that one-third of American hospitals have evaluated robot technology for drug dispensing, but fewer than 10 percent have made such a purchase.

Building Revenues

The Internet can be a revenue pipeline and cash accelerator. Currently, the lag time from a doctor visit to the filed and adjudicated claim to the receipt of data (and revenues) by the provider is two months (Crozier 2000). Ideally, providers should get treatment authorization, claims submission and review, and electronic payment within 48 hours.

HIPAA may be a key enabling factor in promoting electronic commerce in healthcare. Newly promulgated federal regulations for HIPAA are intended to standardize and facilitate electronic transactions. Although many providers are confused about the new HIPAA requirements, the move toward universal standards for transactions between providers and plans is inevitable. The new regulations currently have a two-year implementation timetable, with exceptions for small health insurers and rural hospitals (however, AHA is arguing that the two-year implementation deadline be extended to three years for all providers).

Outsourcing

In the "build-versus-buy" equation, more healthcare providers may choose to purchase their information system and technologies through outsourcing arrangements. Financial pressures from Medicare budget cuts and managed care contracts are compelling managers to reassess outsourcing as a cash-flow and expense reduction strategy. Consultants predict that "hospitals are getting to the point that they don't want somebody to come in and tell them how to do it, they want somebody to do it" (Corrales 2000).

Outsourcing offers a number of advantages to provider organizations, including:

- predictable costs of IS and IT as guaranteed by the vendor;
- enterprisewide assessment of IS and IT needs by the vendor;
- strategic plan for information systems upgrades and new technology;
- access to preferred prices for new technology through the vendor;
- reliance on the vendor to provide all needed management and technical staff;
- shifting of provider IS and IT staff off the payroll, eliminating salaries, benefits, and long-term commitments;
- ability of the vendor to recruit, retain, and flexibly deploy staff;
- access to the vendor's preferred business relationships with major IS and IT suppliers; and
- performance guarantees from the vendor.

In Monroe, Michigan, the Mercy Memorial Hospital recently announced a five-year outsourcing partnership with Superior Consultant. Under the $10 million, five-year arrangement, Superior will systematically upgrade Mercy Memorial's information systems, lead digital technology initiatives, and strive to achieve cost-beneficial performance in the hospital's information systems. Outsourcing enables a community-based hospital like Mercy Memorial to have access to the latest tools, technologies, and technical staffing assistance at a lower cost and greater performance efficiency than the hospital could have likely achieved on its own.

Provider Intranet Networks

Building intranets between a hospital and its physicians may be one of the most effective physician-bonding strategies of the paperless hospital. Hospital-sponsored intranets, which connect physicians for minimal up-front or subscription fees, are proving highly popular. Reliance on a hospital-sponsored intranet can solve many physicians' HIPAA problems, giving them a HIPAA-compliant network and standards for transmitting patient data.

But few physicians are electronically linked with their hospitals. Even among the 100 most-wired hospitals and health systems, accord-

Table 5.1: Physicians' Online Access to Clinical Information

Online Access to Data	100 Most Wired (%)	All Respondents (%)
Access patient data	29	13
View radiology results	26	12
View lab results	25	12
View pathology results	24	12
Decision support*	18	9
Lab order entry	13	5
Pathology order entry	12	5
Pharmacy order entry	12	5
Radiology order entry	12	5

*For example, clinical pathways.

Source: Solovy (2000, pp. 33–34).

ing to the *Hospitals & Health Networks* survey, only about one-third provide clinicians with online access to patient data (Solovy 2000). One in four of the most-wired institutions offers laboratory or radiology reports online, but many hospitals cannot handle online order entry from doctors' offices (see Table 5.1).

The Wisconsin Health Information Network (WHIN) is a provider-sponsored health information system that links hospitals, doctors' offices, laboratories, employers, pharmacies, and insurance companies (Klein 1999). The WHIN network uses Claimsnet, a proprietary online transaction processing service, to batch and speed up medical claims electronically. Network sponsors hope to achieve the 20 percent savings predicted by consultants at Boston-based Arthur D. Little. A pilot study of the WHIN system at the University of Wisconsin–Milwaukee showed that healthcare providers can achieve substantial savings: physician practices can save $17,000 to $68,000 per year based on an average cost reduction of $2.62 per information request via WHIN. Hospitals in the WHIN study achieved savings of $5.10 per information request, generating $400,000 to $1.1 million per year, depending on the volume of data requests.

The Internet is a prime example of a "disruptive technology"—an innovation that revolutionizes markets and industries but can fail because highly regarded companies are unable to accept or adopt it (Christensen 1997). This results in the innovator's dilemma for established firms that face new competition that is better, faster, and cheaper than the current market-leading products. Personal computers from Apple were a disruptive technology to IBM's dominance in mainframe devices. General Motors lost more than half of its market share to Japanese compact automobiles. Health maintenance organizations were disruptive technologies to conventional health insurers such as Prudential, Travelers, and Metropolitan, three of the five largest independent insurers who have all exited the health insurance market. In the near future, "Internet appliances" such as Palm Pilots and cellular, Internet-enabled telephones may become disruptive technologies to personal computer makers.

Disruptive technologies often get their start in market niches too small or unprofitable for large firms to serve. New competitors are unknown firms operating out of low-cost industrial parks, staffed by entrepreneurs working for stocks and bonuses instead of salaries and benefits. They represent unfair competition to established firms that have high overhead costs and an established technology to defend. The recent history of the dot-com companies is filled with examples of new firms whose business model is based on disruptive technology. The $150 billion U.S. telecommunications marketplace has been profoundly shaken by Internet start-ups. Telephone companies, once the bastion of the last surviving monopolies of the twentieth century, are now being threatened by Internet service providers at every business line of established giants like AT&T and GTE. Competition is global with $700 billion in communications revenues up for grabs in a battle of "high stakes and no prisoners" (Ferguson 1999).

Many Internet enterprises will fail, but a few will succeed, ultimately displacing long-established companies that could not respond with lower costs or improved processes. Dallas, Texas–based Paymentech, Inc., provides an example of success using disruptive technology.

Many consumers have been reluctant to reveal their credit card information on the Net, and Paymentech, in response, became a specialist in Internet-based "card not present" transactions and is now the largest U.S. processor of Internet e-commerce by consumers, with clients including Amazon.com, AOL, and Lands End. The company's growth exceeds 15 percent annually, and its profit margins are substantial.

Healthcare providers are now closely watching the future of high-profile dot-coms such as drkoop.com, PlanetRx, Healtheon/WebMD, and HealthCentral. Most have lost their high-flying share prices, which enabled a blizzard of stock-based acquisitions. Now the dot-coms must face the challenge of sustaining growth, demonstrating profitability, and taking significant market share—and revenues—away from mainstream companies. Within the next two to three years, dot-com upstarts will merge and consolidate with established firms such as EDS, GTE, and Premier.

MANAGING TRANSITIONS TO EMERGING TECHNOLOGIES

If managers can understand and harness these forces rather than fight them, they can in fact succeed spectacularly when confronted with disruptive technological change (Christensen 1997, p. xix). But managing the transition to the emerging technology or idea is never easy. Disruptive technologies may have lower profit margins for producers and require substantial adaptation costs by consumers who initially do not want or cannot use them. Customers who have large sunk-cost capital investments in the dominant technology now face the customer side of the innovator's dilemma—when to accept and purchase the new technologies. Hospitals and health systems that have invested millions of dollars in distributed networks of powerful personal computers will soon face the dilemma of potentially displacing or replacing these hard-wired computer networks with small, wireless, handheld electronic medical record devices.

The establishment of "alpha customers" and "beta sites" is a strategy for becoming part of the leading edge of change by creating strategic business relationships with companies testing new products and systems. Market leaders are those who never stop innovating and are recognized as the first to introduce new technologies to their customers. Organizations committed to continuous innovation are willing to share information with suppliers, customers, and even competitors. Houston's MD Anderson Cancer Center shares its clinical protocols with other cancer specialists over the Internet and gains three of four patients from outside the greater Houston market.

Large organizations are often criticized as being slow to adapt, but they do possess some substantial advantages during times of technological change. Very large hospitals and health systems can leverage their hundred million dollar is and it budgets to invest in new technologies. Capital is the key to investment in technologies that can reduce the marginal costs of administrative or clinical services. The advantage of size ("scale") is that economies of scale repeated over and over can translate into million dollar savings. Smaller facilities that are not part of integrated systems often lack the capital for technology investment or do not have the scale to gain real economic benefits.

Health organizations can move more quickly up the learning curve by scanning for emerging applications outside the boundaries of the health industry. Innovation is rampant in many other sectors today. Healthcare organizations can anticipate new tools and products by carefully watching other leading-edge companies. Devices that may become the wireless electronic medical record of tomorrow are already on display, based on the latest electronic communications gadgets emerging in the marketplace (Mount 2000). Samsung has a watchphone, just like cartoon dectective Dick Tracy's. Palm Pilots are being outfitted with global positioning systems to locate anything, anywhere. Ericson's "future tool" is a handheld personal digital assistant that incorporates voice recognition, a rotating video camera, and a "Bluetooth"-enabled earpiece that eliminates the need for a cord between phone and headset. The Anoto pen scans text as it is being written and transmits it to a computer or cell phone. Finally, the "I-mode" is a rapidly growing set of wireless applications for cellular telephones with wireless connections to the Web.

The real innovator's dilemma is whether to stand pat with current technology, with all its sunk costs, installed bases, and staff familiarity, or to continuously adopt and adapt to new technologies incrementally as they become available, at the cost of semicontinuous disruption and year-in, year-out capital investment.

The difference between the market leaders and followers may not be obvious in the first year or two, but by the third year, the innovative organization will begin to gain the cost or strategic advantages, or both, of technology innovation over those organizations who would not, or could not, change. Market consumption and behavior is changing rapidly and fundamentally: more people use Yahoo daily than view the most popular television show. The leaders in tomorrow's Internet-advanced marketplace will be those "incumbent" organizations that have the courage (and capital) to become the insurgents who will make the new trends and reinvent their businesses.

LOOKING FORWARD

E-solutions are the leading edge of a wave of technologically driven change which will ripple across every aspect of healthcare's clinical and administrative processes. Some of these innovations will come from the private business sector, such as supply-chain management or online health plan enrollment. Other new solutions will be specific to healthcare, for example, electronic physician order entry. Progress in the introduction and diffusion of e-solutions will be facilitated—or impeded—by the organization's culture and willingness to change.

Rosabeth Moss Kanter of the Harvard Business School, in her recent book, *e-Volve: Succeeding in the Digital Culture of Tomorrow*, identifies ten reasons why the digital transformation is resisted (Kanter 2001, pp. 256–57): (1) loss of dignity, fear of embarrassment; (2) loss of control when not involved in decisions; (3) excessive uncertainty and feeling uninformed; (4) automatic defensiveness when there is no chance to get ready; (5) does not fit mental model; (6) concerns about competence; (7) disruptions to "normal" work activities; (8) additional things to do, and no time to do it all; (9) memories of other, past problems; and (10) anger that change will inflict pain, create losers.

Resistance to change in the digital era is normal and not unexpected. It is natural for workers and managers to feel concerned about their personal computer literacy and competency when processes are automated. Busy physicians and nurses may resent the time needed to learn new capabilities, such as electronic medical records and computerized order entry. The digital transformation is a transitional and generational issue. Baby Boomers who comprise the majority of today's doctors, RNs, and middle managers have not grown up with computers, as have the "Gen X" younger workers who will replace them within 20 years. The acceptance of e-solutions must be planned, nurtured, and incentivized if healthcare is to fully realize their benefits. The labor shortages in healthcare offer an opportunity to introduce technology solutions which can free up time for caregiving and improve patient safety. For the electronic revolution to ultimately succeed, healthcare's top management must have an unwavering commitment to the e-transformation and model the behavior needed to encourage staff and caregivers to utilize these new electronic tools.

STRATEGIC IMPLICATIONS

Healthcare provider organizations can identify and harness the potential of disruptive technologies in a number of ways.

Scan the Techno-Horizon. Continuously monitor the marketplace for new technology applications. Travel to conferences and seminars on e-health, e-commerce, and information technology given by associations such as HIMSS and Comdex. Subscribe to online news services that showcase new technologies in healthcare, for example, Superior Consultant's "e-briefing" on WebMD and Arthur Anderson's "Knowledge Space."

Become Tech-Savvy at the Senior Management Level. Challenge every member of the senior management team to become expert in the emerging technologies that support their administrative responsibilities. Internet-based technologies are bringing new solutions in such areas as financial transactions (CFO), recruitment (vice president for human resources), alternative service providers and data warehouses (CIO), risk management or error reduction systems (COO/vice president for clinical affairs), and enterprisewide decision-support systems (CEO).

Create a Culture of Constant Improvement. One of the most widely read business magazines today is the upstart *Fast Company*. Articles are slanted toward industries with intense competition, continuous innovation, rapid product development cycles, and aggressive cost cutting. As mentioned throughout this book, the health industry tends to lag behind other sectors in adoption of new technologies; a culture of constant improvement can provide a first-mover advantage to those hospitals, health systems, or medical organizations that take the lead in innovation.

REFERENCES

Baisden, H. 2000. "Harris Sees Internet Health Information Seekers Increasing Markedly Since 1998." *AHA News Now,* August 14, p. 2.

Christensen, C. 1997. *The Innovator's Dilemma: When New Technologies Cause Great Firms to Fail.* Boston: Harvard Business School Press.

Coile, R. C., Jr. 1999. "HIPAA: The 'Next Y2K'." *Health Trends* 12 (4): 1–12.

Collen, M. F. 1998. "A Vision of Health Care and Informatics in 2008." *Journal of the American Informatics Association* 6 (1): 1–5.

Corrales, S. 2000. "Memorial MDs Can Browse Clinicals." *Inside Healthcare Computing* 10 (5): 7–8.

Crozier, M. 2000. "Implementing an Internet-Based Reporting System." *IT Health Care Strategies* 2 (3): 8–9.

Danaher, K. 2000. "Using the Internet to Improve Daily Operations." *Health Management Technology* 21 (2): 40.

Davis, S., and C. Meyer. 1998. *Blur: The Speed of Change in the Connected Economy.* New York: Warner Books.

Downes, L., and C. Mui. 2000. *Unleashing the Killer App: Digital Strategies for Market Dominance.* Boston: Harvard Business School Press.

Egger, E. 1999. "Health Care Use of Internet Faces Both Driving Forces and Barriers." *Health Care Strategic Management* 17 (10): 19–20.

Ferguson, C. H. 1999. *High St@kes, No Prisoners: A Winner's Tale of Greed and Glory in the Internet Wars.* New York: Times Business/Random House.

Garets, D. 2000. "Back to the Future: Experts Predict IT Changes and Developments Most Likely to Affect Health Care in 2000." *IT Health Care Strategist* 2 (2): 1–6.

Haugh, R. 2000. "To the Rescue: New Tools to Prevent Medical Errors in the Workplace." *Hospitals & Health Networks* 74 (4): 44–48.

Kanter, R. M. 2001. *e-Volve: Succeeding in the Digital Culture of Tomorrow.* Cambridge, MA: Harvard Business School Press.

Kilbridge, P. M. 2000. "Urging Providers to Embrace the Web." *MD Computing* 17 (1).

Klein, J. 1999. "Wisconsin Health Information Network Offers Internet-Based Transactions." *IT Health Care Strategist* 1 (9): 11.

Martin, C. 2000. *Net Future: The Seven Cybertrends That Will Drive Your Business, Create New Wealth, and Define Your Future.* New York: McGraw-Hill.

McCormack, J. 1999. "The Top 10 Ways the Internet is Changing Healthcare IT." *Health Data Management* 7 (12): 34–39.

Mjoseth, J. 2000. "Back to the Future: Experts Predict IT Changes and Developments Most Likely to Affect Health Care in 2000. *IT Health Care Strategist* 2 (2): 1–6.

Morrisey, J. 1999. "Just a Click Away." *Modern Healthcare* 29 (39): 5–7.

Mount, I. 2000. "No, It Won't Actually Make Coffee ..." *E-Company* 1 (2): 110–11.

Ruffin, M. D. 1999. *Digital Doctors.* Tampa, FL: American College of Physician Executives.

Schonfeld, F. 2000. "He's Got the Whole Web in His Hands." *E-Company* 1 (2): 105–14.

Schwartz, P., P. Leyden, and J. Hyatt. 2000. *The Long Boom: A Vision for the Coming Age of Prosperity.* Reading, MA: Perseus Books.

Shortell, S. M., et al. 2000. *Remaking Health Care in America,* Second Edition. San Francisco: Jossey-Bass.

Siwicki, B. 1999. "Diving into the Internet." *Health Data Management* 7 (7): 89–90.

Solovy, A. 2000. "Is an E-Commerce Gap Emerging Among the Nation's Hospitals?" *Hospitals & Health Networks* 74 (4): 30–41.

CHAPTER SIX

Web Strategies: The Internet and Customer Relationship Management

KEY CONCEPTS: • *Internet empowerment* • *Health-seekers* • *E-prescriptions* • *P2P* • *Customer relationship management* • *Content partners*

INTRODUCTION: Searching for health information is now the number one reason consumers log onto the Internet. Some 52 percent of almost 100 million Internet users went online for health information last year, according to the Pew Foundation's Internet and American Life Project. The availability of health information on the Web is empowering consumers and fundamentally affecting the patient-physician relationship. "Health seekers" are a new category of Internet users who are searching online for disease-specific information, health advice, and guidance in selecting providers. Internet-savvy providers and health plans are responding to the rapid rise in health seekers by developing Internet-based customer relationship strategies.

"THERE IS ABUNDANT evidence that use of the Internet has played a role in revolutionizing the more than $1 trillion health care industry in America. Doctors, hospitals, health maintenance organizations (HMOS), insurance companies, and Internet firms are using the Internet to retool the business of medicine."

—*Susannah Fox et al. (2000, p. 8)*

The online revolution in healthcare has begun. Consumers in record numbers are flocking to the Internet for health information and advice. According to a recent study by the Pew Internet and American Life Project in Washington, DC, some 52 million Americans sought health information on the Web last year (Fox et al. 2000). Health is now the number one reason consumers log on to the Internet. On a typical day, five million Americans can be found on the World Wide Web seeking health and medical information. More Internet users have sought medical information (55 percent) than have shopped online (47 percent), looked up stock quotes (44 percent), or checked sports scores (36 percent).

Healthcare providers are responding to these electronic demands. Joliet, Illinois–based Provena Saint Joseph Medical Center is partnering with eKiosk to place stand-alone Internet workstations in hospital waiting areas so patients can check their e-mail and browse the hospital's web site (Raphael 2001).

The e-health population is growing at roughly twice the rate of overall Web users (see Figure 6.1). Almost one-third of Web-savvy "health seekers" go online weekly, and another 30 percent pursue health information monthly for themselves or family members. Americans are spending 34 hours—almost a day and half—each month on the Web (Nielson/Net Ratings 2000). The latest Internet usage statistics for a typical Web user show an average of 62 Internet sessions per month, with 19 at home and 43 in the office. Web users are browsing 2,250 pages per month, averaging a half-hour per session.

The availability of health information on the Web is empowering consumers and fundamentally affecting the patient-physician relationship. A 1999 survey by Yankelovich Monitor found that half or more of Americans were not satisfied with the availability of their doctors, nor were they satisfied with the amount of time they spent with their physicians (Fox et al. 2000). Only 3.7 million Americans have e-mailed their doctors' offices, but 33.6 million say they would like to do so, according to the Cybercitizen Health 2000 study by Cyber Dialogue, an Internet market research organization (Gratzer 2000).

Patients are also becoming more involved in managing their health with online information. Some 25 percent of Internet health seekers

Figure 6.1: E-Health Population Growing Faster than Total Online Users (Users in Millions)

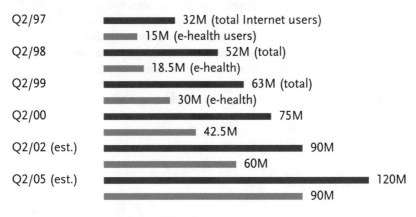

Q2/97 32M (total Internet users)
       15M (e-health users)
Q2/98 52M (total)
       18.5M (e-health)
Q2/99 63M (total)
       30M (e-health)
Q2/00 75M
       42.5M
Q2/02 (est.) 90M
              60M
Q2/05 (est.) 120M
              90M

Source: Cyber Dialogue (2000, p. 1).

are asking their doctors for specific brand-name prescriptions based on information they received from the Web. Surprisingly, 91 percent of health seekers have health insurance. Despite concerns about the digital divide between rich and poor, health seekers come from all income levels and ethnic groups, unlike users of online auctions or banking, who are more likely to be white and affluent.

Internet health seekers are not just shopping for doctors or hospitals. More than 40 percent of those who searched the Web for health information report that the search affected their decisions about the following:

- whether to go to the doctor;
- how to treat an illness;
- what questions to ask their physicians;
- how to take care of themselves, improve self-health;
- information about medications; and
- how to improve ways to get health information.

Figure 6.2: Demographic Profile of Internet Health Seekers

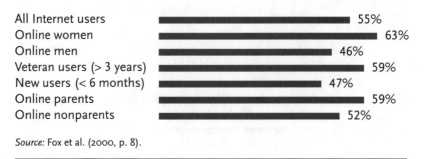

All Internet users	55%
Online women	63%
Online men	46%
Veteran users (> 3 years)	59%
New users (< 6 months)	47%
Online parents	59%
Online nonparents	52%

Source: Fox et al. (2000, p. 8).

Who uses the Web for health information? The short answer is women and baby boomers. Predominantly, Internet health seekers are women (see Figure 6.2). Two in three American women with Internet access have used the Web for health information, whereas only one in two men have done so. On a typical day, 59 percent of health seekers on the Web are women. The highest users are between ages 30 and 64. Two-thirds of women boomers between ages 30 and 49 have gone online for medical information. The Pew Project's data show that long-time users of the Internet are even more likely to have relied on the Web for health purposes: 59 percent of those with three years of Internet experience versus 47 percent of those using the Internet only within the past six months. With little guidance from their physicians, 80 percent of health seekers say they found the sites themselves, and 60 percent reported that the site they got information from was one they had never heard of before beginning the search (O'Neill 2000).

HOSPITAL WEB SITES BECOME UNIVERSAL CONNECTORS

Virtually all of America's 5,000 hospitals offer web sites to connect with consumers, physicians, suppliers, health plans, and their work-forces. The average hospital spends $99,000 per year on managing and expanding its web site, according to a national survey by *Inside Healthcare Computing* (IHC 2000). Budgets for Web-related activities doubled from $45,000 in 1999, with 63 percent of hospitals expanding their Web spending. Many hospitals are still not convinced that a web site is worth the investment. Only 47 percent of hospitals responded "definitely yes" when asked if they received a return on their investment.

Hospitals are still divided about how to manage their web sites. One in two hospitals put their public relations (PR) department in charge of Web communications, whereas 44 percent of hospitals put their information systems department in charge. The choice of which department takes responsibility makes a big difference. Budgets for web sites were a skimpy $18,000 per year under PR leadership but jumped to $62,857 annually when managed by IS.

Connecting with consumers is the most popular use of hospital web sites today, but that is changing. Physician communication will be much more important in the future, health information managers predict in the 11th annual HIMSS Leadership Survey. The initial emphasis on B2C is broadening to including supply-chain relationships, payer communications, patient online scheduling, and health assessment (see Figure 6.3). Many hospitals—59 percent—had not put any physician services online. Hospitals that experimented with sending medical news from WebMD to their physicians have found little physician response.

RETOOLING MEDICINE FOR THE INTERNET AGE

The Web is reinventing the practice of medicine and providing a whole new dimension to the doctor-patient relationship. Patients feel empowered and are taking more control of their health and medical treatment decisions. Consumer empowerment is likely to please pharmaceutical manufacturers, as more than half (54 percent) of regular health users of the Internet report that they ask their doctor about a prescription drug after visiting health web sites (Cyber Dialogue 2000). One in two health seekers say they have urged a friend or family member

Figure 6.3: Hospital Web Site Survey

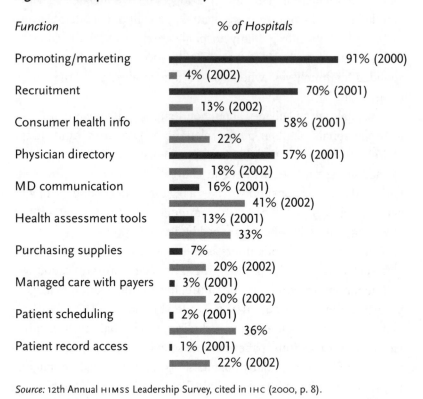

Function	% of Hospitals
Promoting/marketing	91% (2000)
	4% (2002)
Recruitment	70% (2001)
	13% (2002)
Consumer health info	58% (2001)
	22%
Physician directory	57% (2001)
	18% (2002)
MD communication	16% (2001)
	41% (2002)
Health assessment tools	13% (2001)
	33%
Purchasing supplies	7%
	20% (2002)
Managed care with payers	3% (2001)
	20% (2002)
Patient scheduling	2% (2001)
	36%
Patient record access	1% (2001)
	22% (2002)

Source: 12th Annual HIMSS Leadership Survey, cited in IHC (2000, p. 8).

to see a physician, and 50 percent say they made a treatment decision after checking for health information on the Web (see Figure 6.4).

Physician acceptance of the Internet is growing. The percentage of doctors using the Web doubled between 1997 and 1999, according to data from the American Medical Association (Mills 1999). Many more physicians have put their offices online; 79 percent of doctors now work in Internet-enabled offices, according to the AMA (Hsih 2000a). Among doctors who have Web-enabled offices, 62 percent have created a practice or personal web site. Despite these encouraging trends, more than 50 percent of physicians actively discourage Internet use in their offices as "wasted time." According to a recent survey by the American

Figure 6.4: Actions Taken by Consumers After Health Site Visit

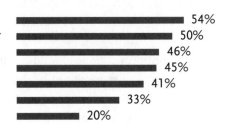

Consumer Actions	Percent of Internet Users
Asked doctor about an Rx	54%
Urged friend/family to see doctor	50%
Altered diet/exercise habits	46%
Made treatment decision	45%
Visited doctor	41%
Taken Rx more regularly	33%
Purchased OTC medicine	20%

Source: Cyber Dialogue (2000, p. 4).

Medical Association, 54 percent of doctors use the Internet in their office, whereas a similiar survey by Deloitte Consulting and Cyber Dialogue found only 24 percent of physicians using the Web in their office (*AMA News* 2001).

Physician resistance is a significant barrier to online medicine. Doctors may be slow to accept the World Wide Web, but consumers are not; the practice of medicine will now be in an open-information environment. Internet-savvy doctors are responding by giving their patients "e-prescriptions"—guiding them to specific health web sites to learn more about treatment options or the management of disease. More than half of all doctors would use e-mail with their patients if they were reimbursed, according to a recent survey by AMA's Medem Internet network (Hsih 2000a). Only 10 percent of doctors communicate with patients using e-mail today. For another use of the Web, the Harvard Medical School recently announced it was creating a new web site, TheAnswerPage.com, for physician continuing medical education (*PR Newswire* 2001). The site's corporate partners will provide educational grants to Harvard for content development, and TheAnswerPage's education programs are free to physicians.

The professional medical establishment also recognizes that the Internet is changing the environment of medicine. Last year, the American Medical Association and six leading medical organizations founded Medem, a physician-sponsored Internet network for doctors and their patients, and recruited Dr. Nancy Dickey, past president of the AMA, as Medem's editor-in-chief. This year, 13 medical societies and the American Medical Association announced a set of principles for physician-to-patient (P2P) Internet communication (Hsih 2000b):

- P2P communications should occur within the context of an existing physician-patient relationship.
- P2P should not be used for emergency situations.
- P2P communications must be private, confidential, and secure.
- Doctors are responsible for diagnosing, prescribing, educating, and advising.
- The Internet is an appropriate venue for requesting health information, clarifying treatment plans, and releasing medical records.
- Some patient situations will require face-to-face evaluation with a physician.
- All participants in P2P communications should use the best available techniques to authenticate identity.
- The physician should make every effort to provide the best, most authoritative clinical information to supplement P2P communications.

FINANCIAL WOES COULD LEAVE FEWER CONTENT PROVIDERS

For the once high-flying dot-com companies, this is "the era of realism," according to Dr. Thomas Linden, an e-health consultant and author of *Tom Linden's Guide to Online Medicine* (Cross 2000, p. 2). Linden believes that e-health is not the solution to America's healthcare dilemma but is simply going to make the existing inefficient healthcare system more effective. Some of the current disillusionment with e-health is due to the volatile stock performance of commercial sites such as drkoop.com and WebMD. Wall Street observers predict that the crowded e-health sector is due for consolidation into a few national firms with brand-name recognition, viable business models, and growing revenues. To survive, a number of e-health companies may merge with other businesses, such as insurance companies, pharmaceutical manufacturers, medical product suppliers, or retail drug chains.

For example, MedicineOnline.com has had to shift its market strategy completely to try to do just that (Heimoff 2001). After starting as a medical content site for consumers, the sinking fortunes of drkoop.com demonstrated that the company could not make money on content alone. In March 2000, after losing much of its venture capital, MedicineOnline switched to a controversial new business—online medical auctions. Through its web site, consumers can find physicians and negotiate a price for a medical procedure. The process is legal, but controversial, and is already being attacked by physician organizations in California as dangerous and unethical. Currently, MedicineOnline does not charge for the service, but it plans to add a consumer surcharge in the future.

Some Internet companies have diversified their offerings to attract both B2B and B2C business and consumer revenues. HealthCentral.com, based in Emoryville, California, is both an online pharmacy and a health information content provider. Although HealthCentral's online pharmacy business has been slow to grow, its content services are attracting a number of hospitals and health systems, including Tenet and Catholic Healthcare West (Heimoff 2001). Providers are attracted to HealthCentral because Dr. Dean Edell, whose radio healthcare program is syndicated to 400 stations, is a cofounder of HealthCentral. The company offers its healthcare organization customers tie-ins to drive business to HealthCentral's online pharmacy for prescription drugs, over-the-counter medications, and vitamins. HealthCentral hopes its provider partnerships can lead physicians to tell their patients "go to this web site" for health information, which can lead to online purchasing of HealthCentral products.

HOW TOP WEB SITES ATTRACT CONSUMERS

America's leading health-related web sites reveal how they attract consumer "eyeballs" and "unique visitors." Hint: you do not have to run an ad during the Super Bowl. Most of these strategies are cheaper and better (Flory 2000a).

- *Use experts and celebrities.* Sports figures, movies stars, and politicians ... an old market strategy works again. WebMD enlisted the help of Muhammed Ali, Lance Armstrong, and Dr. Dean Ornish to host online chats, participate in online communities, and appear in WebMD commercials. Lance Armstrong, a recovered cancer patient and three-time winner of the Tour de France, has also participated as a guest columnist in WebMD's health advice column for *Readers Digest.*
- *Give rewards.* Think "frequent flyer rewards." Some health web sites offer prizes to users, such as computers or PDAS, awarded at random to site visitors. Other web sites give discounts on health services or products, such as DrugEmporium.com's 25 percent savings coupons.
- *Promote around holidays and special events.* The American Heart Association's web site makes special plans around Valentines' Day. The new year puts many consumers in mind to improving health, diet, and fitness. Another top attraction for the holidays is a segment that addresses coping with depression.
- *Conduct a survey.* Many sites are finding that survey poll results are an attractor. The Managed Care Information Center features the "question of the month," recently focusing on healthcare executives' opinions on capitation. WomenOutdoors.com polled its site visitors on their post-holiday plans and discovered that 60 percent vowed to be more active in the new year.
- *Create a crisis center.* Pick a problem and dedicate a site to it. PlanetRx launched a "Cough & Cold Advisor" service on its site just in time for flu season. KidsHealth.org offers tips on the prevention and treatment of colds.

In Pennsylvania, the Children's Hospital of Philadelphia (CHOP) is investing $16 million over the next three years to become a "national leader in e-medicine," according to the *Philadelphia Business Journal* (2001). The university-based children's hospital launched its web site in 1996 but felt that it lacked brand identity. To give the site a turbo boost, the hospital has hired 26 full-time employees and 20 contract employees. Content will be provided by Greystone but tailored to fit CHOP's image and market strategy. CHOP's web site will also generate revenue by reselling content to other sites, as well as developing "off-site" disease management programs. The site will feature simple graphics to shorten downloading time for Web users and an expanded library of pediatric health articles. Families can browse for disease information and participate in online support-group communities.

All this content is delivered with no advertising. The web site is designed as an access center, with online scheduling, physician referrals, and online inquiries. Hospital officials predict the site will break even by the second year through content sales and increased volume, which the site drives to the hospital.

CONSUMER PRIVACY AND HIPAA

The issues of security, confidentiality, and privacy of electronic medical records and Internet transaction will drive healthcare providers and plans to upgrade their total data systems. Final regulations for HIPAA were released by the Clinton administration in late 2000, almost a year after preliminary regulations were issued amidst controversy and criticism. Compliance with HIPAA could cost the health industry over $20 billion in the next two years, according to a study for the American Hospital Association, a figure substantially higher than the cost estimates of the federal government.

Under the final regulations, doctors and hospitals will need to obtain written consent from patients before releasing medical information, even for routine transactions like submitting claims. Both electronic and paper medical records are included in the regulations, although the original legislation only focused on electronic records. Some industry observers predict that the new Bush administration will want to review the regulations released by the outgoing Clinton administration and that some changes in the regulations may result.

Most hospitals and medical offices have waited to see the final regulations before moving to assess their HIPAA needs. In the meantime, healthcare information consultants have mounted extensive provider education programs to bring hospitals and doctors up to speed on how to comply with the complex new regulations.

Consumer and provider organizations have been quick to criticize the new federal privacy rules as inadequate. Some 50,000 comments were received. Providers and health plans complained that the new HIPAA regulations were another "unfounded federal mandate" that would add administrative expenses with no recognition or payment for the cost burden. Consumer organizations expressed concern that law enforcement agencies could access patient records without a court order. Consumers were also not given the right to sue if their records were accidently released. A hospital in the Northwest recently had an unintended Internet disclosure of patient information, which has stirred consumer fears about privacy. The leak reinforced the concern that "if a patient's medical information is compromised, we can have a disaster on our hands," states John Lowenbergh, M.D., president of Medical Data Solutions (Glasheen 2000a, p. 1). As a result, computer security experts see trouble ahead. Doctors are not used to treating medical records as though they are secret government documents, and many physicians are paying scant attention to HIPAA in their own office systems so far.

Several excellent online resources provide the latest information on HIPAA, including the following:

- Aspe.hhs.gov/adminsimp/Index.htm—The administrative simplification page of the Department of Health and Human Services (DHHS) includes regulations, implementation guides, and timetables for publication of proposed HIPAA rules.
- Ahima.org—The American Health Information Management Association (AHIMA) has two excellent privacy documents, including "Analysis of the HIPAA Electronic Transactions and Code Sets" and "Recommendations to Ensure Privacy and Quality of Personal Health Information."
- Epic.org—EPIC is a public-interest research center, the goal of which is to focus public attention on consumer privacy and First

Amendment issues. The site includes news, policy statements, and a number of resources and guides.

- Csrc.nist.gov—The Computer Security Division of the National Institute of Standards and Technology is an agency of the Department of Commerce's Technology Administration. The site offers an index of information on computer vulnerabilities, as well as information about advanced encryption standards and security best practices.

Internet users are worried about the safety and security of personal health information that is shared online, according to a recent survey by the California Healthcare Foundation and the Internet Healthcare Coalition (Glasheen 2000b). Based on a poll of more than 1,000 consumers, the survey found that over 75 percent of those seeking health information on the Web are "concerned" or "very concerned" about the sites with which they have registered. Consumer confidence rises if the site has been recommended by a physician, publishes a privacy policy, offers users a chance to see who can access profiles, and allows users to make choices about information use. Tie-ins with insurers or pharmaceutical firms made consumers nervous, out of concern that private information might be used for marketing or advertising. The new HIPAA regulations are intended to allay such consumer concerns by forcing providers to get advance permission to share data and compelling disclosure of any commercial relationships.

NINE INTERNET STRATEGIES FOR CUSTOMER RELATIONSHIP MANAGEMENT

The e-health war for the consumer is on. Providers and health plans are beginning to compete to become the consumer's most trusted web site and portal for managing the patient's or enrollee's health needs. Making life easier for the customer will dominate as an overall trend in healthcare next year, and the Internet will play a major—and integrated—role, predicts Jay Toole, national director of E-Health, Cap Gemini Ernst & Young (Cross 2000, p. 2). In the "post e-health" era, the concept of independent commercial web sites for health consumers is evolving into an integrated model that utilizes the Internet as a customer relationship management strategy for providers and health plans. The core of the strategy is building value for customers, which will translate into vendor loyalty, repeat business, and future demand and will include communicating with consumers.

Health plans and providers have a lot of catching up to do in this area. The Internet can help, but Web initiatives must be part of a global customer relationship management strategy.

Internet companies have scaled down their ambitions to create "killer aps" (Downes and Mui 2000). Still, in the past five to seven years, the Internet has fundamentally changed many businesses and created new ones. By making it easier for people and the devices they use to find, share, and add to their information base, the Internet has created an open market in the truest sense. Availability of low-cost Internet access devices and essentially free information has energized consumerism. Healthcare has become one of the most popular information sets on the Web, evolving rapidly from an online medical dictionary and physician directory into a rich, complex database of increasingly detailed information about diseases, diagnostic and theraputic options, and five-star-rated sources of treatment.

With that in mind, nine strategies for customer relationship management on the Web follow.

1. Provide Disease-Specific Information

The majority of consumers come to the Web looking for information on the management of specific diseases in an effort to assist themselves or family members in managing health conditions. Allergies are the number one topic researched, followed by cancer and heart disease (see Table 6.1). The e-health market is recognizing women as the top users and realigning its sites to provide information that spans the continuum of diseases, disorders, and conditions that are unique to, more serious for, or more prevalent in women (Bernard 2000). Sites that target women offer information, interactive communications, and subsections on women's diseases and conditions. In the future, many

Table 6.1: Top Health Conditions Sought on the Internet

Disease	Online Seekers (%)
Allergies	37
Cancer	35
Heart disease	29
Diabetes	26
Digestive disorders	24
Arthritis	24
High cholesterol	22
Migraine	20
Asthma	19

Source: Cyber Dialogue (2000, p. 3).

women-oriented health web sites will also offer specific products for women's health conditions, including over-the-counter drugs, home diagnostic kits and testing devices, medical supplies, and durable medical equipment.

2. Consider Content Partners

More providers and plans will rely on outside content partners to supply increasingly detailed and sophisticated health information packaged for Internet users. Fewer sources of Internet health content may be available in the future: the number of dot-com health content suppliers is already shrinking, and further consolidation is likely by mid-2002. Of today's estimated 20,000 health-related web sites, approximately 15,000 are content sites (Glasheen 2000b).

During 2000 and into 2001, increasing horizontal consolidation has occurred among the commercial Internet health content suppliers. For example, Mediconsult.com, a physician portal, has recently purchased a competitor, Physicians Online, in an attempt to gain significant "eye-share" in the content space. "Vertical" integration and consolidation has also increased among Web health content providers, with firms taking on additional functions such as e-commerce, communications and connectivity, and Web-based healthcare services (Glasheen 2000c). E-health firms are increasing their search for revenues, moving beyond advertising and sponsorships to include online newsletters, product sales, and telemedicine.

3. Create Interactive Sites

Health-related web sites sponsored by hospitals, doctors, and health plans will be increasingly interactive in the next two to five years. Most provider-sponsored sites are "infomercials," which offer consumers one-way ability to communicate through e-mail. Consumers want quick-response or real-time Internet communication for appointment scheduling, preadmission paperwork, and testing results. To address this, information technology experts predict that providers and insurers will add a host of new features on their web sites that foster two-way communication with consumers.

At California-based Kaiser Permanente, health plan members will have the ability in 2001 to schedule appointments and refill prescriptions in real time. The HMO has designed an Internet-enabled process that links consumers through the Kaiser web site directly into the scheduling and pharmacy systems—the same information systems that Kaiser employees use (Cross 2000). This will be a major improvement over the past system, in which Kaiser members had to e-mail the plan and wait for a response. Kaiser Permanente Online, started as a pilot project in 1996, now has 324,044 registered users on its companywide web site (*Wall Street Journal* 2001). The password-protected site allows users to e-mail queries to nurses and pharmacists for advice, as well as join doctor-monitored online health discussion groups and personalized health assessments.

A few hospitals are going well beyond two-way Internet communications to assist patients in creating online personal electronic medical records. In Kansas City, Missouri, the Cerner Corporation is partnering with Winona Health, which operates 99-bed Community Memorial Hospital (Haugh 2000). The project, Winona Health Online, creates a personalized home page for each consumer. Patients access their home page through the Winona Health portal, and health encounters such as doctor visits, prescriptions, hospitalizations, and lab results are logged and tracked. Secure connections ensure privacy, and the service is available on a 24 × 7 basis. Future plans include health risk assessments and personal health improvement plans. The Winona project links a number of community-based providers together, which project sponsors call a mini-CHIN, a concept introduced in the 1990s that struggled to gain acceptance and sponsorship in practice.

4. Utilize Mass Customization

Customer relationship management begins with marketing efforts based on databases that are "mined" for information. From such a starting point, an Internet-enabled marketing program can use the Web, telephone, direct mail, or traditional advertising as mass customization tools to reach potential consumers. Mass customization is the ability to reach one consumer at a time on a personal level, utilizing individual and unique information. Providers find that direct mail is preferred by most customers, but use of the Internet is increasing. Few hospitals or medical groups have made more than superficial uses of their patient databases (clearly, under the new HIPAA federal regulations, providers cannot utilize confidential patient data). However, providers can take advantage of historical databases of service utilization and patient preferences to target consumers, for example, by age, sex, and geographic location. Companies like Solucient and CPM (Customer Potential Management) Marketing Group offer proprietary systems for constructing marketing databases and pinpointing target consumers, as well as providing market research (Weber 2000).

5. Employ Physician Linkages

Internet-hip physicians are beginning to change the way medical professionals interact with patients. As doctors build web sites, they will forgo fancy "plug-ins" of disease information from content providers and stick with simple but interactive sites, predicts Dr. Michael

Rothschild, a pediatric ear, nose, and throat specialist in New York, whose book, *Building and Implementing Physician Practice Web Sites,* will be published by the American Medical Association in 2001 (Cross 2000, p. 5). Doctors will offer their e-patients opportunities to complete online questionnaires, and some physicians will also open their appointment books for online scheduling. One-third of physicians are already using the Internet multiple times each day, according to a recent survey by *Modern Physician* (VHA 2000). The top three physician-used web sites are Medscape, WebMD, and drkoop.com, according to a recent survey by BioInformatics, Inc. (Flory 2000b).

Physician referral is one of the most visited areas of provider web sites. With labels like "Find a Doctor," online physician directories typically offer background and credentials information, office hours, address and telephone, and special services. More sophisticated physician directories include special services and areas of specialization, and some also offer e-mail communication. Few physician sites can offer online scheduling, but more group practices are planning to make it available in the next 12 to 24 months. Resistance among some physicians to online directories can still be found, however (Steele 2000). Some physicians express security concerns about electronic publishing of photographs or personal information. Doctors may be reluctant to publish their office's e-mail address for fear of being overwhelmed with patient e-correspondence.

6. Leverage Branding

Branding gives leverage in a field where many health-related web sites are struggling to build or buy brand reputation. Many Internet companies such as WebMD have spent millions of dollars to establish brand-name recognition. Some Web-based firms, such as e-HealthAxis, which sells health insurance online, have spent much of their venture capital on advertising, and others never survived long enough to build a brand. LaurusHealth.com has spent years establishing its brand, even though it has been backed by a strategic business relationship with Irving, Texas–based VHA, one of the largest hospital group purchasing organizations in the nation. Successful Internet firms like Amazon

.com also are still spending heavily on media. It takes five years to fully establish a new brand in the minds of consumers.

But many healthcare organizations have well-known brands that can be transformed into Web addresses, including some of the nation's best-practices sites such as MayoClinic.com, Allina.com, and advocatehealth.com (Flory 2000c). Mayo recently shifted its brand strategy for Oasis.com to using its better-known Mayo Clinic name on the web site. The Mayo experience suggests that use of the provider organization's name in creating web sites will capitalize on brand equity and keep advertising costs down.

7. Exploit the Ratings Game

Consumers will use report cards to select providers, predicts *Futurescan 2001*, a new environmental forecast prepared by the American Hospital Association's Society for Healthcare Strategy and Market Development (Coile 2001). Hospitals are now playing the ratings game, jockeying for position to be a top 100 or five-star facility. Consumer rankings and report cards provide comparative information to consumers when they select a hospital or doctor. Achieving top 100 hospitals status from Solucient is one of the most highly sought designations in the field. Top 100 hospitals average 22 percent higher occupancy, employ 18 percent fewer staff, experience 16 percent better quality, and are consistently more profitable than peers (Reeder 2000). For the year 2000, the top 100 had an average total profit margin of 8.7 percent, in comparison with the average hospital, which squeaked by with a 1.9 percent bottom line. In the latest 2000 ratings, the eighth year for the top 100 rankings, only one hospital—Boston's 650-bed Brigham and Women's Hospital—has been selected among the best of the best for all eight years (Lovern 2000).

Winning a five-star rating from HealthGrades.com, a Lakewood, Colorado–based market research firm, signifies that a hospital's clinical care ranks among the best of the best. HealthGrades.com provides online ratings of providers through its web site, and ratings are based on Medicare's MEDPAR data, supplemented by data from 16 states that also maintain databases on all inpatients (HealthGrades.com 2000).

Just like hotels and restaurants, HealthGrades.com provides ratings up to five-star recommendations on six dozen popular specialty services, such as open-heart surgery and joint replacement surgery. The top-ranked hospitals can purchase the marketing rights to their five-star ratings, and many use them for advertising to promote the services. Ratings cover 5,000 hospitals, and HealthGrades.com also offers unrated profile information for 400 health plans, 600,000 physicians, 7,800 home health agencies, 60,000 chiropractors, 150,000 dentists, 75 birth centers, and 3,000 hospices.

8. Develop Strategic Business Relationships

Hospitals and physicians can expand their reach through affiliation with commercial and nonprofit web sites. Partnerships can increase traffic to both sites, providing a value-added service for consumers who only have to double-click to access the related site. Among commercial Web companies, PlanetRx is actively seeking tie-ins with other sites to boost the number of visitors (Heimoff 2000). (Wall Street has taken its eyes off PlanetRx because of its slow revenue growth.) The company is in the process of becoming licensed in every state and is seeking recognition as a pharmaceutical services partner by HMOs and health insurers. In the interim, PlanetRx has focused on growing revenues through sales of over-the-counter remedies and products. Through PlanetRx's "Affiliates" program, participating dot-coms offer PlanetRx on their sites. In return, they earn 15 percent of all sales, as well as cash bonuses for every new customer referred to PlanetRx through the site. PlanetRx has also created a "Partners" program, constructing strategic alliances with IBM, Barnes & Noble, and E-Trade, which is intended to boost traffic in both directions (Heimoff 2001).

9. Use Outsourcing

Hospitals are turning to outside firms for their Internet services, for design as well as operation of their web sites. As consumers become more demanding and Internet competition intensifies, many hospitals do not have the in-house resources to expand their health information content or the information technology expertise in web site development and management because they lack expertise or find recruiting and retaining webmasters difficult.

However, outsourcing may be risky as well. The outside firm will need strategic direction and oversight. In some cases in which the outside firm fails to perform, contractual dissolution can be costly and time consuming. Disputes over ownership of intellectual property— the web site content—have occurred. Sadder but wiser hospitals recommend several steps to structure an outsourcing relationship:

- Be aware of potential legal problem areas, such as contracts, disclaimers, and ownership of intellectual property.
- Use an e-commerce attorney to draft the contract with a Web developer, content provider, or Web operator.
- Know the strengths and weaknesses of the outsourcing firm, and check references.
- Identify the outside firm's policies on intellectual property, patent issues, and trademark insurance.
- Set a realistic budget, discuss the issue of cost overruns in advance, and check the accuracy of the firm's cost estimates with other clients.
- Continue to evaluate the site and include in the contract a provision to use focus groups to evaluate consumer satisfaction.

LOOKING FORWARD: A REALISTIC OUTLOOK FOR WEB STRATEGY

The Internet changed the rules of competition and created a new economy. But too many Internet companies tried to grow their business with marketing strategies that defied the laws of mathematics. As one Wall Street observer notes, "dot.com marketing has been driven by a giant leap of faith—the equivalent of a seven-year-old leaping from a tree house to prove gravity is wrong" (Kirsner 2001, p. 44). E-companies were willing to spend more than the lifetime value of a customer;

that strategy was obviously not sustainable. Now the digital economy is facing marketing realities and is moving toward a model that sparks the desired action: getting someone to visit a site, subscribe to an e-mail newsletter, or make a purchase (Kirsner 2001, p. 44).

The e-health marketplace is still in a period of turmoil, and consolidation is accelerating the pace of change among commercial firms like drkoop.com, HealthCentral, HealthGate, Medscape, and WebMD. Healthcare provider organizations must sort out winners and losers as they seek partners to outsource content and web site operations. The good news is that health consumers are flocking to the Internet for health advice and information. But very quickly, today's sophisticated Internet users will tire of the regurgitated content that is offered by many provider-sponsored web sites. Providers need a holistic Internet marketing strategy that is part of their broader strategy of customer relationship management.

The Internet is a two-way communications channel. Providers need to know who their consumers are and talk to them, advises John Halleck, president of CPM, to provide the information needed to achieve better health and wellness (Weber 2000). Only those providers that use a long-term investment strategy are likely to transform their customer relationships in a way that will increase their total volume while improving consumer satisfaction.

One of the fundamental differences between for-profit and non-profit organizations is the expectations for growth. Wall Street wants high growth and continuous expansion, so investor-owned companies must demonstrate 15 to 20 percent annual growth and return on investment. For a time in 1998 and 1999, Wall Street investors abandoned their usual insistence on business growth, accepting other non-economic indicators such as "traffic" and "eyeballs" as indicators of future volume and potential revenues. Eventually, the investors demanded real revenues and profits, and the stock market punished drkoop.com, WebMD, PlanetRx, and other healthcare dot-coms that could not produce significant revenues or reduce their losses.

Nonprofit organizations are not required to grow at such a hectic pace. Incremental growth provides an opportunity to evaluate whether

Web strategies are working and to cut back or refocus Web investments if the strategies are providing adequate pay-back.

A growing number of hospitals, health plans, and suppliers are recognizing the need to partner with other firms in creating and sustaining Internet-based customer relationship management strategies. The attraction of a strategic business relationship is the opportunity to utilize the skills, expertise, market recognition, and infrastructure that the partner brings. Thus, affiliations are flourishing among dot-coms. The business model in partnering is changing from up-front fees to after-the-sale revenue sharing. Partnerships with organizations are comprised of shared business and market goals, not just a customer-vendor relationship. Incentives for the partnership or affiliation should be incorporated in the partnership agreement to reward business goals such as increased customer volume or revenues.

Interest in outsourcing content and technology is growing. In many situations, outsourcing can be the low-cost strategy for most hospitals, physician groups, and health systems. For any provider organization or health plan that intends to offer more than simple directories of services or doctors, outsourcing content and technology is the best way to implement its offerings. The Internet's "e-space" is rapidly consolidating to a small number of commercially viable companies that can provide healthcare information, expert advice, commerce, and connectivity. Few Web-based companies have the expertise or hardware to operate their own Internet sites. Even fewer have the capability to expand service offerings, upgrade content, or improve the interactivity of their site. The complexities involved in HIPAA compliance add another reason for healthcare providers to outsource the development and maintenance of their web sites.

The ultimate lesson about the Internet and consumers relates to the concept of customer value. Consumers may visit a site once out of curiousity or because they were pulled over with a hot-link. But consumers will only return if the web site offers value and meets customer needs. Many health seekers on the Web are sophisticated frequent users, and consumer expectations are evolving toward greater quality coverage and quality content, predicts Joyce Flory, coeditor of *Internet*

Healthcare Strategies (Flory 2000a). She advises potential paperless organizations to improve the interactivity, depth of content, and features that facilitate the consumer relationship, such as online appointment scheduling and access to lab and radiology results.

STRATEGIC IMPLICATIONS

As healthcare organizations begin to expand their entry-level web sites into Internet market strategies, what can providers, health plans, and suppliers learn from the dot-com roller coaster? If history is what we call our mistakes, the lessons of the dot-coms should be very instructive. Much may be learned from the past five years of the digital economy.

Integrated Web Strategy. Too many dot-coms mistakenly thought *the* Internet was *the* strategy. Driving eyeballs and unique visitors to the web site were the goals, with little consideration for what to do with the customers once they were on the site. The lesson: Web strategy should be a component of the organization's overall market strategy. It is not the strategy.

Realistic Business Model. The business journals have been filled with stories of dot-coms caught in a death spiral of rising expenditures to acquire customers and too few revenues to cover marketing costs. The result was predictable. Continuing losses by the e-firms accelerated the "burn rate" until the investment capital was spent. The lesson: Build a business model on realistic premises addressing increases in volume, utilization, attracting new customers, customer retention, and market share.

Investment for the Long Term. Among investors, "invest for the long term" is the first rule, but it is easily forgotten when major swings are occurring in the prices of publicly traded companies. Last year, when Wall Street momentum disappeared in the Internet sector, many companies collapsed in a matter of months. The lesson: Know the costs and revenues of the Web-induced incremental volume, and make reasonable business judgments on how much to invest in Web-based marketing.

REFERENCES

AMA News 2001. "More Physicians on the Internet, but Not for Professional Tasks." Cited in "News Tidbits," February 8, p. 1. [Online news brief.] Southfield, MI: Superior Consultant.

Bernard, S. 2000. "Women's Health and the Web." *Healthcare Leadership Review* 19 (5): 2.

Coile, R. C., Jr. 2001. *Futurescan 2001: A Millennium Forecast of Healthcare Trends 2001–2005,* pp. 1–36. Chicago: Health Administration Press and the American Hospital Association.

Cross, M. A. 2000. "What's Next? Experts Look Ahead to 2001." [Online news story.] *Internet Healthcare Magazine,* December 8, pp. 1–6.

Cyber Dialogue. 2000. "Cybercitizen 2000." Market Research Report, August, p. 1. New York: Cyber Dialogue.

Downes, L., and C. Mui. 2000. *Unleashing the Killer App.* Boston: Harvard Business School Press.

Flory, J. 2000a. "What Consumers Expect: Faster, Better, Closer." *Internet Healthcare Strategies* 2 (10): 1–7.

———. 2000b. "Web Winners: Medscape Ranks as Number One Physician Portal." *Internet Healthcare Strategies* 2 (3): 14–15.

———. 2000c. "The Top Portals' Hottest Promotion Strategies." *Internet Healthcare Strategies* 2 (3): 7.

Fox, S. et al. 2000. *The Online Health Care Revolution: How the Web Helps Americans Take Better Care of Themselves,* November 26, pp. 1–23. Washington, DC: Pew Internet & American Life Project.

Glasheen, J. 2000a. "Security and Confidentiality." *Medicine on the Net* 6 (11): 1–4.

———. 2000b. "Survey Watch: Internet Users Wary of Health Privacy Breach." *Internet Healthcare Strategies* 2 (3): 15.

———. 2000c. "The Four Healthcare Internet Site Segments Are Consolidating and Converging." *Healthcare Marketing Abstracts* 15 (3): 4.

Gratzer, C. 2000. "Cyber Dialogue: The Future's Bright for Online Health Industry." [Online news story.] Nua Ltd., August 24.

Haugh, R. 2000. "A Wired, Healthy Community." *Hospitals & Health Networks* 74 (7): 40–42.

Healthgrades.com. 2000. "Hospital Report Cards Methodology White Paper: 2001 Analysis" (1997–1999 data), August 22, pp. 1–3. Lakewood, CO: Healthgrades.

Heimoff, S. 2000. "Marketing and Health B2C Revenue Promise." Part 1. COR Healthcare Market Strategist 1 (9): 1–2, 11–15.

————. 2001. "Marketing and Health B2C Revenue Promise." Part 2. COR Healthcare Market Strategist 2 (1): 5–9.

Hsih, C. 2000a. "Latest Research Reveals that Half of Physicians Interested in Using E-Mail with Patients If Reimbursed." [Online press release.] American Medical Association, November 6, pp. 1–2.

————. 2000b. "Thirteen of the Nation's Leading Medical Societies Recommend Best Practices for Harnessing the Internet to Empower the Patient-Physician Relationship." [Online press release.] American Medical Association, November 28, pp. 1–2.

Inside Healthcare Computing (IHC). 2000. "Hospitals Are Pleased with Own Web Site Efforts; Many Spend Little." *Inside Healthcare Computing* 10 (11): 7–8.

Kirsner, S. 2001. "The New Lure of Internet Marketing." *Fast Company* FC42: 44–46.

Lovern, E. 2000. "Reaping Healthy Profits: 100 Hospitals Manage to Come Out On Top Even in Year Plagued by Financial Ills." *Modern Healthcare* 30 (51): 36–40.

Mills, R. J. 1999. "AMA Study Finds that Physician Web Use Has Doubled." [Online news release.] American Medical Association, December 6, pp. 1–2.

Nielson/Net Ratings. 2000. "Traffic Patterns: October 2000 Internet Usage Stats." [Online news story.] November 21, pp. 1–2.

O'Neill, J. 2000. "Health Care Online and in the Third Person." *New York Times*, December 19, p. D8.

Philadelphia Business Journal. 2001. "CHOP: Revamps Web Site to Become National Leader in E-Medicine." Cited in "News Tidbits," February 2, pp. 1–2. [Online news brief.] Southfield, MI: Superior Consultant.

PR Newswire. 2001. "Sticky Website Creates New Way for Medical Industry to Market to Physicians and Conduct Market Research." PR Newswire. Cited in "News Tidbits," March 15, p. 2. [Online news brief.] Southfield, MI: Superior Consultant.

Raphael, S. 2001. "Internet Kiosk Unveiled in Illinois Hospital's Main Lobby." [Online news brief.] *Superior Health,* December 15, p. 1.

Reeder, L. 2000. "Implementing Performance Improvement in Health Systems." *Healthcare Leadership & Management Report* 8 (7): 1–7.

Steele, G. W. 2000. "The Next Generation Healthcare Organization Web Site." *Internet Healthcare Strategies* 2 (3): 9–11.

VHA. 2000. "Health Care 2000: A Strategic Assessment of the Health Care Environment in the United States." Irving, TX: VHA.

Wall Street Journal. 2001. "Information Therapy May Help Treat Patients." Cited in "News Tidbits," February 2, pp. 2–3. [Online news brief.] Southfield, MI: Superior Consultant.

Weber, D. O. 2000. "CRM: When Marketing Gets Personal." *Healthcare Leadership Review* 19 (5): 1.

CHAPTER SEVEN

Outsourcing: A Better, Faster, Cheaper Solution for Technology Management

KEY CONCEPTS: *ASPS • BSPS • Customer relationship management • Data centers • Executive steering committees • Gainsharing • Hosted applications • Performance-based contracting • Virtual data exchange*

INTRODUCTION: Outsourcing is the "better, faster, cheaper" solution for managing the digital transformation of hospitals and health systems. Relying on outside firms for help in upgrading healthcare IT systems is a growth market that is starting "now": outsourcing is one of the new killer apps. Many firms are utilizing outsourcing as a strategy for focusing on their core businesses. Outsourcing arrangements today are based on mutually set performance expectations between client and vendor. Gainsharing between the provider organization and the outsourcing firm recognizes the mutual responsibility of both parties to make an outsourcing relationship work. In tomorrow's wired world, healthcare providers need e-partners with expertise, networks, applications, hardware, and the technology toolkit to build digital business and clinical solutions.

"SOMETIMES THERE ARE too many skills needed, too many skill-hungry projects to complete, too many specialized operations to support, and not enough skilled professionals to go around. In the healthcare industry, where money is chronically tight, it doesn't make sense to hire people with all the collective skills needed for all purposes, even if they could be found and hired. The answer for some organizations is to bring in outside expert help, not just to advise and consult on how to do the information systems tasks, but to help do the work."

—*Walt Zerrenner, CIO, New York–Presbyterian Hospital and Health System (Pasternak 2001, p. 8)*

Outsourcing is the "better, faster, cheaper" solution for managing the digital transformation of hospitals and health systems. Relying on outside firms for help in upgrading healthcare information technology (IT) systems presents an immediate growth market. According to Gartner Dataquest's five-year forecast, the worldwide market for outsourcing finance, accounting, and information technology management could soar 300 percent, from $12 billion in 1999 to $37.7 billion in 2004 (Business Wire 2001a). Gartner's optimistic forecast assumes that new technologies and Web delivery of applications will accelerate the adoption of outsourcing as a way of increasing operational efficiency, gaining competitive advantage, and creating shareholder value. In healthcare, the Meta Group predicts that expenditures for IT outsourcing will increase from $200 million in 1999 to $3 billion by 2003 (Anderson 2000).

A number of factors are driving healthcare organizations to adopt IT risk-sharing outsourcing alternatives:

- IT skills shortages are widespread; 37 percent of IT positions are still open.
- Healthcare ranks last in IT wages among the nation's nine largest industries.
- Healthcare is unable to compete for IT salaries with other industries.
- IT project failure rate is high, estimated at over 70 percent.
- Turnover of chief information officers and IT staff with high-demand skills is rapid.
- Change in information technology, infrastructure, and applications is continuous.
- Complex new federal HIPAA regulations for information privacy must be implemented within three years.

Outsourcing is one of the "killer apps of the new information-based economy" (Downes and Mui 1998). Many firms are utilizing outsourcing as a strategy for focusing on their core businesses. Outsourcing noncore functions to vendor-partners, such as web site maintenance, managing off-site data warehouses, and building and maintaining information networks with physicians, enables senior management to concentrate on the organization's core competencies, critical business activities, and high-value customers. Outsourcing also offers healthcare providers the opportunity to acquire and distribute knowledge without the time and cost of producing that knowledge internally, for example, Web content, consumer health information, and disease management.

Outsourcing can work for big and small clients. Large IDNS can outsource multiple functions, preserving their capital and using best-of-breed outsourcing vendors for specialized functions. Small clients—solo hospitals and small systems—can be "thin clients," whose in-house information technology is limited but has access to powerhouse IT infrastructure through the outsourcing vendor (Hochstadt and Lewis 1999). Outsourcing could account for 20 percent of hospital budgets by 2002, according to a recent survey by VHA of Irving, Texas, and Michael F. Corbett & Associates of Boston (HFMA 2000). Hospital spending on outsourcing rose by 20 percent between 1999 and 2000, the VHA study reported, and *Modern Healthcare*'s annual outsourcing survey showed 16 percent growth during 1998–99 (Shinkman 2000). Outsourcing options range from supplemental staffing with outside personnel to strategic alliances and joint ventures with business partners. The shift to outsourcing was most evident in organizations with more than $500 million in annual revenues and covered a broad range of clinical, financial, IT, and support operations. Outsourcing of IT functions is one of the most popular applications, representing 18 percent of all outsourcing arrangements, according to the VHA survey.

MANY WAYS TO OUTSOURCE

Outsourcing is a highly flexible approach to the installation, maintenance, operations, and management of information technology. Some of the outsourcing options include:

- alternative service providers (ASPS);
- staff leasing;
- interim CIO or other management;
- technology installation and maintenance;
- IT operations;
- time sharing or equipment sharing; and
- help desk functions.

Vendors are unbundling functions for IT outsourcing, which is contributing to their rapid growth. Provider organizations can choose the functions they wish to contract out, while maintaining other IT functions internally. More than a dozen key IT functions are being outsourced today by hospitals and health systems across the nation, according to a national survey by the Meta Group (Anderson 2000) (Table 7.1), and many providers are turning to more than one vendor to provide specialized expertise. In Fort Worth, Texas, the JPS Health Network, a division of the Tarrant County Hospital District, contracts with InfoHealth Management Corporation of Chicago, which coordinates the activities of four outside contractors with 31 employees working on JPS projects (Pasternak 2001). Their diverse responsibilities under InfoHealth supervision include installation of new hardware and software applications, setting up and maintaining secure local and intranet networks, and responding to calls for service. JPS has only one employee on its IT payroll—the CIO. InfoHealth manages all other workers in the multifirm outsourcing arrangement, changing the skill mix on an as-needed basis as the JPS information system evolves.

BENEFITS OF OUTSOURCING

The tide is turning toward outsourcing IT. According to a recent industry study by the Cutter Consortium, more than 50 percent of surveyed companies reported they were outsourcing more functions than they did a year ago (Cutter Consortium 2001). Positive experiences with prior outsourcing arrangements are contributing to an expanded outlook. So are shortages of key IT personnel. Encouraged by their

Table 7.1: Top Outsourcing Areas in Healthcare

IT Function	Surveyed Hospitals (%)
Software development, installation, support	21
Network design and support	20
PC/desktop maintenance and support	19
Data center operation	14
Consulting and contract programming	10
Hardware maintenance and support	9
Billing/financial system operation, support	8
Technical services	7
Telecommunications support	7
PC/desktop acquisition and installation	6
Help desk	6
Management	5
WAN design and support	4
PC/desktop training	3
Clinical system operation and support	2

Source: Anderson (2000, p. 4).

positive history with outsourcing vendors, more companies are willing to turn over a growing array of key IT functions to outsourcing partners (see Table 7.2).

Cost savings are a primary reason for outsourcing. In Michigan, the Detroit Medical Center (DMC) signed the first $1 billion, ten-year healthcare outsourcing contract in the fourth quarter of 1999 (Anderson 2000). CareTech Solutions of Farmington Hills, Michigan assumed all risks associated with the successful installation of all applications purchased by DMC. In year one, the outsourcing vendor guaranteed a 15 percent decrease in IT costs, along with long-term savings of $100 million, which are projected over the ten-year contract.

When markets change rapidly, or when time costs money, speed is a critical success factor (Information Access Company 2000). More

Table 7.2: Five Leading IT Functions for Outsourcing

Application development	52%
Hardware maintenance	47%
Training	45%
Web design	40%
Application maintenance	35%

Source: Cutter Consortium (2001, p. 6).

organizations are looking to access skills by buying them instead of growing them organically. Companies see an outsourcing provider as being able to help them speed up process improvement. Stan Davis and Christopher Meyer, coauthors of *Blur: The Speed of Change in the Connected Economy* (1998), argue that information technology and Internet connectivity are changing our perceptions of time, space, and mass. High-speed connectivity has led to the "death of distance" and exploded the reach of consumers and suppliers. Outsourcing makes sense for a capital-intensive activity like information systems management, with its rapid obsolescence of technology and high personnel turnover. Outsourcing offers healthcare providers immediate access to skills, infrastructure, and specialized expertise, with the benefits of reducing capital costs and shortening time to market.

Complying with HIPAA is another good reason for outsourcing IT functions. Given the short timetable—two years—and the complexity of the new federal regulations, many provider organizations will spend millions of dollars on consultants and new staff hires to become compliant with HIPAA before October 2002 for electronic transactions and April 2003 for consumer privacy regulations. New York University–Presbyterian's CIO Walt Zerrenner asks, "Do you really want to hire and train staff, and then audit all the applications they install for HIPAA compliance? I don't think so" (Pasternak 2001, p. 4).

OUTSOURCING CUSTOMER RELATIONSHIP MANAGEMENT

Customer relationship management (CRM) is one of the hottest trends in the new economy. CRM shifts the focus from the company to the customer with the goals of increasing brand awareness and brand loyalty, increasing volume, obtaining premium pricing, and enhancing customer retention. The market for CRM is predicted by Kennedy Information to grow from $8.6 billion in 1999 to $44.4 billion five years thereafter (Kennedy Information 2000). Applying information technology and the Internet to the customer interface can create seamless, customized relationships. The CRM model requires extensive databases, systems development, data analysis, integration of information across the organization, and implementation of personalized Web experiences by customers.

Two software vendors dominate the CRM market: Siebel Systems and Oracle. Siebel started with call center automation and expanded into sales force automation, customer service, and channel building. Oracle dominates the market for data warehousing but has expanded into other aspects of customer relationship management. The largest e-tailers use CRM extensively. Amazon.com analyzes past purchasing patterns and suggests new offers for books, music, or electronics based on past customer preferences recorded in their database. Outsourcing CRM avoids the capital costs of building large data warehouses and takes advantage of vendor-built software for interactive web sites and personalizing patient-provider communications. Health-related web sites are now being constructed for increased interactivity, tapping into their data repositories to build personalized patient sites. In the future, healthcare providers will build IT-enabled customer relationship strategies, which begin with universal registration. CRM strategies can be used for health education of the "worried well" population, as well as disease management for the chronically ill. Within the next two to five years, IT-savvy hospitals and health systems will apply CRM to customize every service and setting utilized by their patients and assist patients who want to maintain a personal electronic medical record.

Table 7.3: Reasons CIOs Are Skeptical of Outsourcing

Not cost-effective	41%
Too expensive	25%
Efficiency or service concerns	18%
Prior negative experience	11%
Privacy and security concerns	9%
Lack of high-quality vendors	9%
Insurance and risk-related concerns	2%

Source: Anderson (2000, p. 2).

INTERNAL OPPOSITION TO OUTSOURCING

The benefits of outsourcing may be easier to sell to CEOs than to chief information officers. Skeptical CIOs cite a number of reasons they are opposed to outsourcing, according to a survey by Stamford, Connecticut–based Meta Group (Table 7.3) (Anderson 2000). Not listed in Table 7.3 is job security; one reason CIOs may fear the arrival of an outside firm is the possibility of the outsourcing vendor replacing the existing CIO with a manager of its own. In the post-outsourcing environment, CIOs may also fear a loss of managerial authority and flexibility. Outsourcing contracts are typically subjected to extensive and continuing management oversight against a detailed matrix of performance standards. Paranoia among CIOs is natural; therefore, consultants recommend development of individual staff retention incentives for CIOs and other key IT managers and personnel as part of the outsourcing agreement.

Decision-making power in outsourcing arrangements is shifting from CIOs to executive steering committees (ESCS). One in four outsourcing arrangements is governed by multistakeholder ESCS, which include the CIO and other key managers from the client and vendor organizations. ESCS provide contract oversight and strategic decisions, combining senior-level project managers and consultants from the client organization and the outsourcing vendor. ESCS are commonly found in large, complex outsourcing projects but are expected to become a widely used structure for many outsourcing agreements.

"VIRTUAL" CARE DATA EXCHANGE

An innovative "virtual network" model for data sharing is attracting attention in Santa Barbara, California. With the cooperation of four competing hospitals and their business partners, the "Care Data Exchange" facilitates data sharing on a countywide basis among hospitals, physicians, payers, and the Santa Barbara Regional Health Authority, which operates the local Medicaid managed care program (Morrisey 2001). The local county medical society also backs the concept and is a founding partner. The project was launched with a seed grant of $10 million from the California Healthcare Foundation, founded in 1996 when Blue Cross of California was converted to a for-profit company, Wellpoint Health Networks.

The Care Data Exchange is managed by CareScience of Philadelphia, a consulting firm that specializes in compiling and analyzing clinical data. CareScience and the partners constructed an Internet network and data exchange standards that share data in a multilevel system, which ensures patient privacy. The network is virtual: no central data repository exists, and all participants hold their own data and share only what is needed and authorized. Other regions are considering the Care Data Exchange as a new form of CHIN.

PERFORMANCE-BASED CONTRACTING

Outsourcing arrangements today are based on mutually set performance expectations between client and vendor. Provider organizations contracting for outsourcing services are not willing to trade one set of problems for another. In Indianapolis, three-hospital St. Vincent's Hospitals and Health Services concluded that the quality of their computer support and response to problems was inadequate and sought an outside contractor to manage IT services. St. Vincent's contracted with Daou Systems of San Diego to take over all desktops and to manage installation of a point-of-care information system that links 5,000 devices (Pasternak 2001). In the new arrangement, 15 of St. Vincent's employees were hired by the contractor under a five-year contract. The system pays the contractor on a sliding-fee scale based on 20 performance incentives, which are renegotiated yearly.

Gainsharing between the provider organization and the outsourcing firm recognizes the mutual responsibility of both parties to make an outsourcing relationship work. In a gainsharing arrangement, the parties set goals and share the economic benefits of cost savings and productivity improvements. The concept of gainsharing provides tangible incentives to build a successful and collaborative relationship. Not all performance objectives have an economic dimension, such as user satisfaction, but many aspects of an outsourcing arrangement can be described in terms of economic effects. When the provider organization and the outsourcing firm are successful in achieving economic targets, the relationship is reinforced in a very positive way.

TEN FUTURE TRENDS IN OUTSOURCING

Time sharing of computers was once the most popular form of outsourcing IT services in healthcare. In an extensive market outlook for information technology in healthcare prepared by San Francisco–based Thomas Weisel Partners, analysts predict that, as IT dollars have become increasingly scarce in healthcare, application and business service providers are emerging and beginning to offer healthcare providers an extremely attractive value proposition. ASPS and business service providers (BSPS), representing perhaps the purest evolutionary form of outsourcing, may have unlimited potential in healthcare IT, especially as confidentiality and privacy concerns are being addressed by HIPAA (Hochstadt and Lewis 1999).

Today, vendors offer many outsourcing options, from single-function support to total enterprise IT management and data center operations. The concept of outsourcing now presents a broad continuum of alternatives, which addresses the key issues of staffing, technology obsolescence, and return on investment. Outsourcing is a 24 × 7 solution to many information-based services that must be available on a continuous basis, and this low-cost, highly flexible model is changing the way many companies do business. Outsource Solutions, Inc., of Waltham, Massachusetts, is a virtual company that operates out of 200 square feet of corporate office space, with only one in-house staffer. All of the company's employees work out of home offices, keeping corporate databases and web sites constantly refreshed around the clock across the United States and Europe (Martin 1999).

The following are the key trends in outsourcing for the next two to five years.

1. Bigger Deals

Organizations are increasingly willing to make multimillion dollar, multiyear commitments to outsourcing (Dash 2000). The first blockbuster deal was $1 billion for ten years, signed in late 1999 between CareTech Solutions of Farmington Hills, Michigan, and the Detroit Medical Center, and the trend is expanding. The St. Joseph Health System closed a ten-year, $270 million outsourcing contract with Dallas, Texas–based Perot Systems Corporation, which will provide IT services to the health system's 15 hospitals in Texas and California. In New York, Presbyterian Hospital has concluded a $200 million outsourcing arrangement with First Consulting Group of Long Beach, California, while across town, the St. Francis Health System recently announced another $200 million outsourcing contract with Southern California–based csc and Superior Consultant of Southfield, Michigan.

2. Digital Transformation

The shift from paper to digital records and the migration of many functions to local area networks and the Internet is driving the growth of outsourcing. In Irving, Texas, Jeffrey Hayes, VHA's vice president of business operations, attributes the outsourcing trend on the nonclinical side of healthcare to the "explosion of technology" that heavily affects hospital front and back offices, coupled with the shift from paper to electronic medical records (Shinkman 2000). Paper-based exchanges in provider organizations are extraordinarily inefficient and require multiple and laborious process steps, which drive up costs.

Fragmentation of existing clinical and administrative processes often overwhelms provider organizations and frustrates patients, payers, and suppliers. The concept of the digital marketplace in healthcare envisions a network of providers, payers, vendors—and even patients—sharing analogous information through a centralized server (Hochstadt and Lewis 1999).

3. Outsourcing by Physicians

Outsourcing of core functions in medical offices is growing, especially by larger medical groups. Medical practices are outsourcing functions for cost-efficiency and quality, as well as coping with shortages of technical personnel. Services like coding and billing are becoming highly complicated, and the practices cannot afford errors, which could lead to financial issues or even regulatory oversight. In some markets, local medical societies are playing a role by developing shared-services and practice support organizations or by certifying vendors (Woodward 2000). In central Ohio, a number of physicians and hospitals process their claims through Medibill, Inc. The company provides a complete billing solution from physician charge information to payment processing and collections (Best Company 2001). The physician market is served primarily by a number of smaller niche players, but larger vendors may see the medical group market as a growth opportunity in the future.

In addition, physician use of computers and the Internet is rising rapidly. One-third of physician practices now have a web site, according to a recent survey by the American Hospital Association, and 13 percent of physicians are now using electronic medical records (Hoppszallern 2001).

4. Outsourcing by Health Plans

Hospitals and physicians may be dealing with an outsourcing vendor in their business transactions with health plans. A growing number of HMOs and health insurers are turning to outside companies to provide technology and digital business solutions. In Massachusetts, Harvard Pilgrim Health Care hopes to save $1 to $2 million by outsourcing its behavioral health claims management process to an outside firm, Massachusetts Behavioral Health Partner (Best Company 2001). Utah's InterMountain Health Care (IHC) has recently contracted with TriZetto to provide a managed care administrative system for IHC's one million health plan members in three states (PR Newswire 2001a). The TriZetto system will link 22 network hospitals, 2,500 physicians, and 100 other affiliated clinics.

5. Disease Management

Outsourcing is providing a better solution to the increasingly costly and complex challenge of managing disease. The cost target is huge—an estimated 60 percent of the nation's healthcare spending is consumed by the chronically ill. The cost of caring for the chronically ill is forecast to rise 16 percent, to nearly $600 billion, by 2010 (Hochstadt and Lewis 1999). Disease management programs offer the potential to predict and prevent acute conditions and improve the quality of life for the chronically ill while reducing their overall costs of care. Patients with comorbidities are particularly challenging. The fragmentation of healthcare delivery is a major issue for patients with complex conditions such as diabetes, cardiovascular disease, hypertension, and ESRD.

Commercial disease management programs now cover more than 1.5 million patients (Business Wire 2001b), and more than 75 percent of these patients are identified through pharmacy claims data. Hospitals and health systems are discovering outsourcing can provide the combination of information technology, care protocols, patient education and compliance programs, and personal support mechanisms (Nissenson 2000).

6. Coding

Among hospitals and health systems, coding is becoming one of the most popular areas for outsourcing. An estimated 5 to 10 percent of hospitals now outsource some or all of their coding activities, which could grow to 25 percent, according to MedGroup Corporation of Monument, Colorado (Business Word 2000). Lack of trained coders is one reason for outsourcing to an offsite coding service, but complex payment regulations and the risk of a payer audit are also driving more hospitals to outsource their coding functions. When federal officials began a high-visibility campaign against the widespread practice of "upcoding," many hospitals became very defensive in their coding practices. In fact, many of them today may undercode, and thus undercharge payers. These issues are being successfully addressed by expert coding companies that are applying specialized expert systems to optimize their claims, resulting in improved payment rates, fewer rejected claims, and increased revenues.

7. Co-opetition

Outsourcing's philosophy of collaboration is being expanded to included competitors. When competitors buy into the potential for group benefit, the notion of competition changes, according to Rick Moore, CEO of Tri-Health, a two-hospital system based in Cincinnati (Morrisey 2001). In the highly competitive eastern Ohio market, HealthBridge is a regional outsourcing initiative that involves seven of the leading healthcare organizations. The Internet-based information network delivers laboratory data and other clinical information to hospitals and their physicians. Mercy Health Partners, a six-hospital IDN, estimates they have saved 80 percent of the up-front costs and 40 percent of the ongoing operational costs of the joint-venture network. Automation of physician order entry and rapid communication of test results could save $55,000 per physician per year when utilizing the shared network.

8. Alternative Service Providers

A growing number of provider organizations are contracting with alternative services providers (ASPs), which provide the functionality of a software application without the need to purchase, install, or maintain either software or hardware (Stevens 2001). Applications can be accessed from any computer via the Web, and implementation is very fast. Many ASP-based applications can be operational in days. For example, in New England, Martin's Point Health Care's network of primary care physician practices have contracted with McKesson to provide a confidential Web-based provider-patient intranet, called Practice Point Connect. Pricing and payment procedures are also innovative: ASPS may charge a monthly or annual subscription, or even bill on a per-use basis.

This is a thin-client solution, where the provider organization only needs a network connection and a PC-based workstation. Maintenance costs are bundled in the subscription rate, and no capital cost, depreciation, or equipment or software replacement are required. ASPS offer a valuable return-on-investment proposition because they can reduce a company's total cost of ownership (Hochstadt and Lewis 1999). Forrester Research estimates that the market for branded application outsourcing services in the United States will be $21.1 billion in 2001.

Wall Street analysts Shattuck Hammond Partners add a note of caution about the future of ASPS: even if they are successful, ASPS must struggle through a cultural and financial mine field that has devasted many companies—cannibalizing higher-revenue sales of client-server products in favor of lower-revenue sales of subscription-based ASP software (Scibetta 2000). Computer service providers (CSPS) offer hardware and technical infrastructure on a subscription or per-use basis. These applications are hosted in world-class data centers with high bandwith, recovery protocols, and redundancy capacity. Forrester Research estimates that the market for managed web site hosting in the United States will grow from less than $1 billion in 1998 to $14 billion in 2003. Exemplifying this increased application, four academic medical centers have recently contracted with HealthGate's e-health platform for Web content and hosting (Superior Consultant 2001). HealthGate, which currently contracts with more than 600 hospitals across the nation, will transform the teaching hospitals' static web sites into interactive resources for patients and providers. Features of the Web-hosting arrangement will include customized Web content, interactive health management tools for consumers, and more than 2,200 hours of continuing medical education (CME) for healthcare professionals.

9. Transition Management

Outside companies can be utilized as a strategy for managing transitions in technology. Vendors can take the lead in implementing new software and hardware side by side with the existing system and processes that are managed internally. Outsourcing these technology migrations keep existing systems running while new-era technology is being installed and brought on line (Joslyn 2001). In the Northwest, ACS recently signed an outsourcing agreement to manage the transition of Affiliated Health Services, a two-hospital system, from HBOC to Meditech (PR Newswire 2001b). The migration services include application software implementation and support, hardware management, education, data repository, and an electronic medical record.

10. Long-Term Deals

The lifespan of outsourcing arrangements is growing, as more organizations gain confidence in their outsourcing strategies and partners. The typical outsourcing contract is now at least three years, and in many cases, five years. A few outsourcing deals stretch to ten to 12 years. Recently, the Bank of Scotland and IBM signed a ten-year outsourcing contract, while Rolls Royce and EDS agreed to work together for 12 years (Ward 2000). CEOS may love the financial terms and stability of these mega-deals, but nearly three in four (72 percent) of IT managers are concerned that such long-term arrangements could become obsolete in the rapidly changing environment of information technology.

LOOKING FORWARD: OUTSOURCING MUST BE A GLOBAL STRATEGY—NOT A TECHNOLOGY FIX

The central purpose of e-strategy is to support the core business strategies of the healthcare organization, such as growth, specialization, market share, quality, and customer service. It is not about hardware, software, or the Internet. Those electronic capabilities are not strategy; e-enabled systems and networks are part of the strategic toolkit of management to achieve the goals of the organization, advises Steve Rushing, a senior vice president for Southfield, Michigan–based Superior Consultant (Rushing 2001).

Outsourcing must address the priority business problems of the organization. The scope of IT outsourcing solutions must be as broad as the problems facing the organization. Harnessing the Internet is not a problem—it is a solution, and outsourcing vendors must rethink their approach to match this view. In Phoenix, Arizona, Reginald Ballantyne, CEO of PMH Health Resources, cites the major issues facing his multihospital system, including severe reimbursement cutbacks, managed care challenges, claims payment delays, the search for capital, and the most severe nursing shortage in memory (Crain Communications 2001). PMH is looking for new solutions to building bridges with their physicians, as well as rebuilding public confidence in hospital quality over medical errors.

Outsourcing is the solution to the innovator's dilemma, when new technologies disrupt traditional business relationships and strategies (Christensen 1997). Old-economy companies can partner with firms that have the specialized expertise, hardware, and systems to provide a new set of solutions. In healthcare, outsourcing information technology began with computer time sharing more than two decades ago, before the proliferation of low-cost desktop computers made decentralized computing possible. Technology sharing is emerging again as a solution to network building and maintenance, coping with complex and competing electronic data interchange standards, and moving quickly to comply with the new HIPAA regulations.

The pace of new outsourcing arrangements is gaining momentum, but it could be faster. Provider organizations may find themselves falling behind when health plans and purchasers adopt e-health outsourcing solutions more rapidly. In California's Silicon Valley, a half-dozen high-tech employers are contracting with Healinx, a physician-run start-up company, to operate an e-mail messaging system that will link 2,000 employees with 100 physicians for health information and medical advice (Health Care Advisory Board 2001). The system encrypts and stores all e-mails, and Healinx automatically sends a bill for $20 per Web visit. The employers hope to reduce urgent care and emergency care costs by 20 percent by encouraging patients to use the Internet for health intervention.

Outsourcing Web visits is just one example of the rapid digital transformation of healthcare. In tomorrow's wired world, healthcare providers need electronic partners with expertise, networks, applications, hardware, and the technology toolkit to provide digital business and clinical solutions. Outsourcing has been unbundled, and providers can contract for one solution or for the turnkey management of an entire system. In the make-versus-buy equation, outsourcing offers a range of solutions.

STRATEGIC IMPLICATIONS

Information technology and the Internet are deconstructing traditional business strategy, advise Philip Evans and Thomas Wurster of the Boston Consulting Group in *Blown to Bits: How the New Economics of Information Transforms Strategy*. The Internet opens up global possibilities for new relationships with Web-connected partners (Evans and Wurster 2000).

Culture and Compatibility. At the end of the day, the success of an outsourcing arrangement may have more to do with culture and compatibility than with economic factors. Managing the culture of an outsourcing relationship is important because IT vendors and clients are "joined at the hip" to provide indispensable services. The history of outsourcing is littered with the debris of failed arrangements and broken contracts. According to the Stamford, Connecticut–based Gartner Group, 60 percent of all outsourcing agreements (across all industries) will not be considered successful by management (Joslyn 2001).

Some Problems Cannot Be Outsourced. Outsourcing is not a one-solution-fits-all-problems strategy. Clients who have a simplistic view of outsourcing are often disappointed. Turning over the management of IT problems and walking away will not work. Some healthcare organizations have gone through the contracting-out cycle more than once before settling in with their vendors and determining which services can be best managed inside and outside the organization. Outsourcing contracts must be carefully managed under a joint client-vendor structure.

Supporting the Organization's Global Strategy. A long-term outsourcing partnership will only succeed when outsourcing arrangements are structured in terms of high-priority strategic objectives and core business issues. Cost savings are still important, but so are other strategic goals such as expanding the business, improving skills, improving service, reducing medical errors, and coping with labor shortages.

REFERENCES

Anderson, M. 2000. "Post-Y2K Healthcare Trends: Outsourcing." Healthcare Information Technology Strategies, File 225, pp. 1–4. Stamford, CT: Meta Group.

Best Company. 2001. "Harvard Pilgrim Could Save $2 Million Through Outsourcing." *Best's Review* 101 (10): 112.

Business Word. 2000. "Many Hospitals Now Outsourcing Coding Functions, Seeing Improved Reimbursement." *Healthcare Strategic Management* 18 (12): 4.

Business Wire. 2001a. "Gartner Dataquest Projects Finance and Accounting Outsourcing to Exceed $37 Billion in 2004." [Online news story.] January 4, pp. 1–2.

———. 2001b. "Disease Management in U.S. Now Covers a Broad Range of Chronic Illnesses." [Online news brief.] March 22, p. 1.

Christensen, C. M. 1997. *The Innovator's Dilemma: When New Technologies Cause Great Firms to Fail.* Boston: Harvard Business School Press.

Crain Communications. 2001. "The Business Case for Outsourcing Information Technology." Eye on Info. *Modern Healthcare* (Suppl.), March 5, pp. 1–2.

Cutter Consortium. 2001. "Many Companies Outsourcing IT." *HP Professional.* Cited in Information Access Company. [Online news story.] April 1, p. 6.

Dash, J. 2000. "Hospital Signs $270M Outsourcing Deal." [Online news brief.] *Computerworld,* February 14, p. 4.

Davis, S., and C. Meyer. 1998. *Blur: The Speed of Change in the Connected Economy.* New York: Warner Books.

Downes, L., and C. Mui. 1998. *Unleashing the Killer App: Digital Strategies for Market Dominance.* Boston: Harvard Business School Press.

Evans, P., and T. S. Wurster. 2000. *Blown to Bits: How the New Economics of Information Transforms Strategy.* Boston: Harvard Business School Press.

Healthcare Financial Management Association (HFMA). 2000. "Hospital Spending on Outsourcing Rises 20 Percent." *HFMA Journal* 54 (11): 20.

Health Care Advisory Board. 2001. "Six Silicon Valley Employers Pilot System for 'Email Visits' with MDs." [Online news brief.] March 23, p. 1.

Hochstadt, B., and D. Lewis. 1999. *Bits of Paper to Bytes of Data,* pp. 1–66. San Francisco: Thomas Weisel Partners.

Hoppszallern, S. 2001. "Physicians and the Internet." *Hospitals & Health Networks* 75 (2): 50–54.

Information Access Company. 2000. "Many Companies Outsourcing IT." [Online news story.] *HP Professional,* April 1, p. 6.

Joslyn, S. 2001. "Strike a Balance with Outsourcing." *Modern Healthcare* 31 (40): 31.

Kennedy Information. 2000. "Customer Relationship Management: Consulting's Next Major Wave." *E-Services Report* 1 (10): 1–10.

Martin, C. 1999. *Net Future: The Seven Cybertrends that Will Drive Your Business, Create New Wealth, and Define Your Future.* New York: McGraw-Hill.

Morrisey, J. 2001. "Sharing Expense, Sharing Success." *Modern Healthcare* 31 (26): 26–30.

Nissenson, A. R. 2000. "Doing It Right Doesn't Always Mean Doing It Yourself." [Online news story.] *Managed Healthcare,* December 1, pp. 36–37.

PR Newswire. 2001a. "TriZetto Announces Erisco Facets Licensing Agreement with IHC Health Plans." [Online news brief.] April 19, p. 1.

———. 2001b. "ACS Signs Implementation Services Agreement with Affiliated Health Services." [Online news brief.] April 19, p. 1.

Pasternak, A. 2001. "What's Right for You?" *Modern Healthcare* 31 (9): 8.

Rushing, S. 2001. "E-Strategy." Presentation to the Board, Rush-Copley Medical Center, Aurora, IL, April 24.

Scibetta, J. 2000. *eHealth Revolution: Tiptoeing ON the Tulips,* pp. 1–27. New York: Shattuck Hammond Partners.

Shinkman, R. 2000. "Outsourcing on the Upswing: Healthcare Providers Are Farming Out More Services to Spend Less Money." *Modern Healthcare* 30 (46): 46.

Stevens, L. 2001. "Hosted Applications." *Medicine on the Net* 7 (3): 1–6.

Superior Consultant. 2001. "Leading Academic Medical Centers Choose HealthGate's CHOICE eHealth Platform." News Tidbits. [Online article.] February 8, pp. 2–3.

Ward, H. 2000. "IT Bosses Say No to Mega Outsourcing." [Online news article.] *Computer Weekly,* July 13, p. 1.

Woodward, K. L. 2000. "Physicians Outsourcing More Administrative Tasks." *Business First–Columbus* 17 (5): B3.

CHAPTER EIGHT

Call Centers: Managing Demand to Manage Care

KEY CONCEPTS: *Information therapy • Self-service movement • Triage call centers • Care management algorithms • Demand management • IVR systems • Emergency hotline • Automated appointment reminder • Automated patient scheduling*

INTRODUCTION: Millions of healthcare consumers are joining the information age to obtain medical information and nurse counseling using toll-free telephone call centers and online health advisors. What began a decade ago as marketing-oriented information and referral services, such as the popular "Ask a Nurse" program, have now become centers of highly sophisticated managed care strategies employing the latest telecommunications and computer technology. Call centers can apply "demand management" protocols to advise patients on how to meet their urgent needs for healthcare in the lowest-cost manner. The best call centers in the United States are investing in measuring performance and emphasizing service quality. Medicine's "virtual practice" era is rapidly arriving, with, for instance, primary care providers and specialists only seeing patients in their offices when absolutely necessary and nurse and patient monitoring being conducted the rest of the time from the "electronic physician office," the call center.

"HEALTHCARE HAS JOINED the fast-paced world of self-service .... Health service companies are now aggressively marketing self-care and demand management—providing the resources for healthcare consumers to assume responsibility for their own care to obtain low costs and more efficient use of services.

—Barbara Hesselgrave (1997, pp. 57–58)

Call it "information therapy." Millions of healthcare consumers are joining the information age to obtain medical information and nurse counseling using toll-free telephone call centers and online health advisors. A recent survey found that 77 percent of patients entering the health system would give up a personal visit with a physician if they could get credible, prompt information by telephone or Internet (Barr, Laufenberg, and Stieckman 1998). Today, call centers respond to about 100 million calls per year and cover 35 million managed care enrollees, which could rise 300 percent to 100 million Americans by the year 2000.

Lily Tomlin's comic role on television's "Laugh-In" program as the telephone operator ("One ringy dingy, two ringy dingy") today is being played out as an important managed care cost-control and consumer service strategy, with nurses answering the telephone lines and dispensing health advice (Straub 1998). Hundreds of toll-free "call centers" are operating across the nation, sponsored by integrated delivery systems, medical group practices, health plans, and HMOs. Many triage call centers respond to 2,000 to 5,000 medical inquiries each month, and the numbers are rising rapidly as consumers discover how to use the Internet to access call centers for online health advice. Healthcare organizations are now spending $100 to $300 million per year for hardware and software to equip call centers (Chin 1998). What began as a marketing approach to drive patients into hospitals and doctors' offices has now become a powerful managed care approach to control the costs of care by channeling the demand and use of services. But the ultimate application of call centers in the future may be the coordination of care for high-risk, high-cost beneficiaries of managed care plans, self-insured employers, and Medicare HMOs.

Early call centers focused on consumer marketing, information, and physician referral. Today, sophisticated call centers such as the

Samaritan Call Center of the Samaritan Health System in Phoenix, Arizona, provide an array of cost control, disease management, and marketing functions, including (Barr, Laufenberg, and Stieckman 1998):

- an access gateway to the health system;
- behavior change monitoring;
- chronic disease management;
- community health alerts;
- database marketing;
- health advice and counseling support;
- increased medical compliance;
- insurance claims submission;
- medical news and information;
- nurse triage and telediagnosis;
- patient self-assessment measures;
- physician referral services and appointment scheduling;
- prescription refills;
- provider-patient communications;
- public relations;
- self-health and goal management; and
- telemedicine.

In Minnesota, physicians and nurses of the Family Physicians of Northfield began to extend the application of their practice guidelines to "tele-visits" between patients and the clinic's staff (Millenson 1999). The guidelines were the product of the Institute for Clinical Systems Integration (ICSI), a collaborative effort between the Twin Cities' Buyers Health Care Action Group (BHCAG) and leading Minnesota provider organizations, including the Mayo Clinic. Northfield clinic staffer Nancy Jaeckels, a laboratory technician, began to translate the complex guidelines onto 5" × 8" cards she called "shingles," which were used by the clinic's office and professional staff. In this process, each guideline was broken down into simple steps, and, the emphasis was on prevention. In one pilot project, the care of patients who called the clinic with symptoms of urinary tract infections (UTIS) was managed by a telephone call from a doctor or visit with a nurse. A lab test was given to confirm the diagnosis, and the patient was treated with antibiotics for three days. Cost of care dropped to $39 per UTI case, versus $133 for managing patients with traditional clinic visits.

HEALTHCARE ADOPTS CALL CENTERS FROM OTHER INDUSTRIES

The first modern call center was created in a joint venture between Rockwell International and Continental Airlines some 25 years ago (Durr 1998). Early call centers were designed to generate revenue. Airlines were a logical venue for call centers to sell airplane seats, a highly perishable commodity, with greater efficiency. Today, call centers have been widely adopted for technical support, catalog sales, and customer service. Many companies have discovered that competitive advantage can be gained by providing easy, toll-free access to product information and ordering. In the health industry, call centers are gaining acceptance from hospitals, physician groups, health plans, and patients. Telecommunications consultants Frost & Sullivan of Mountain View, California, estimate that the total U.S. market for call centers will grow 16 percent annually from 1998 to 2004, with total revenues of $10 billion in five years (Frost & Sullivan 1999).

As call centers multiply in the healthcare environment, they are facing new challenges, including competition, profitability, excess capacity, and role definition. In some markets, health plans and provider networks operate competing call centers, which can result in confused consumers being forced to choose among alternative toll-free telephone numbers. A more vexing issue for all call centers that provide care management is determining their ultimate role—cost control or customer service. Among call center managers, the issues of quality, profitability, and turnover are ranked top among their management concerns (see Figure 8.1).

The rapid growth of healthcare call centers has not been without obstacles, and some issues are still to be overcome. A recent national survey found a number of concerns in call center operation and system integration (Krup 1999):

Figure 8.1: Major Issues Facing Call Center Managers

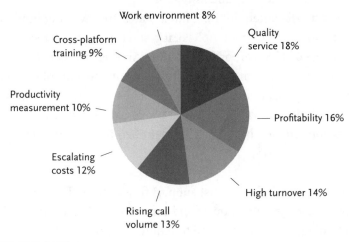

Work environment 8%

Cross-platform training 9%

Quality service 18%

Productivity measurement 10%

Profitability 16%

Escalating costs 12%

High turnover 14%

Rising call volume 13%

Source: Krup (1999)

- cost per person;
- quality service;
- profitability;
- high employee turnover;
- managerial training;
- employee health; and
- workplace environment.

Employee morale and turnover are among the most persistent operational problems experienced by call centers, according to a survey of 300 call center managers by Center Core, a call center furniture maker in Plainfield, New Jersey (Krup 1999). A majority of call centers routinely experience up to 20 percent turnover, one in three centers sees 21 to 50 percent of their staffers depart, and 10 percent of all call centers lose 50 to 100 percent of their staff each year. Outsourcing the management of the call center may become a dominant industry pattern, three of four call center managers predict. And call centers may become virtual, 74 percent of managers forecast, with remote staffing and in-home locations, which could improve job flexibility and morale for call center workers. Voice recognition technology may also improve future efficiency and lower costs.

The best call centers in the United States are investing in performance measurement and emphasizing service quality. A recent survey of 21 major U.S. corporations by the American Productivity and Quality Center (APQC) in Houston, Texas, identified a number of best practices across call centers operating across industries including health, banking, insurance, discount brokerage, and investment services. Among the ten best practices identified in the survey were the following (APQC 1998):

- The call center culture must support front-line staff.
- Upper management support and commitment is critical.
- Technology must support the function.
- Employee loyalty must be engendered and rewarded.
- Structured and focused feedback must be provided.
- Concentration should be focused on a few performance measures.
- Employee needs must be recognized and met.

MANAGED CARE, CONSUMERISM ARE THE DRIVING FORCES

In a growing number of markets, managed care is the driving force behind the explosion of call centers in American healthcare. Rick Stier, president of Health Potentials, a St. Petersburg, Florida–based consulting firm specializing in call centers, observes that managed care has forced a change in focus by call centers from generating revenues through physician referrals to reducing costs and managing the health needs of members (Chin 1998, p. 122).

Health plans and capitated providers have a built-in incentive to hold down health costs. Call centers can apply "demand management" protocols to advise patients on how to meet their urgent needs for healthcare in the lowest-cost manner, such as scheduling a physician appointment for the following day instead of advising the patient to seek immediate care from an emergency room. In call centers operated by health plans and capitated physicians or integrated systems, their demand management programs redirect care to the most appropriate site and the appropriate time to improve cost-efficiency. Medicaid HMOs have discovered that call centers can substantially reduce unnecessary use of emergency care for common illnesses, such as the flu, colds, and earaches. The Oregon Health Plan, the state's managed Medicaid program, contains costs by staffing its call center with 15 inmates from the state penitentiary in Salem, handling 30,000 calls each month (Serb 1998).

The ultimate applications of call center technology may be disease management and health promotion. Managed care organizations must address the health needs and costs of two basic populations: the 10 to 20 percent of enrollees who are at high risk for needing healthcare today, and the 80 to 90 percent who are healthy or may be characterized as the worried well and use only limited health resources now. HMOs and capitated providers have a long-term incentive to put high-risk patients under continuous care management and to promote the health of those who are not (yet) chronically ill.

In California, one of the state's largest HMOs, HealthNet, has established a call center to service commercial, Medicare, and Medicaid HMO enrollees. HealthNet's call center provides telephone-based triage services from registered nurses and offers access to an audio library of two- to five-minute recordings on 400 health topics (Chin 1998). Software from Access Health, based in Rancho Cordova, California, prompts the nurse to ask a series of questions, depending on the patient's complaints and symptoms.

CARE MANAGEMENT ALGORITHMS

Nurse-staffed call centers provide health advice based on protocols developed by physicians and nurse practitioners to manage the most frequently arising consumer health needs. These patient care management guidelines are "algorithms," defined in broadest terms by Webster's Collegiate Dictionary (Tenth Edition) as "step-by-step procedure[s] for solving a problem or accomplishing some end especially by a computer." Earlier seen by doctors as "cookbook" medicine, the possibility of algorithm-generated guidelines being imposed by the federal government decreased when the Clinton health plan collapsed. Now it is the private sector and managed care that are driving the standardization of medical practice. Physicians across the nation are applying their clinical expertise to translating sophisticated medical practice guidelines into decision rules, which nurses can apply when advising patients by telephone or online.

Call center guidelines are continuously updated by incorporating the latest medical literature, as well as the evaluated experience of the call centers themselves, by tracking outcomes and costs of consumers who are triaged and managed by the centers. Phoenix-based National Health Enhancement Systems utilizes experience from its "Micromedex" database to improve guidelines and referrals by its call centers (Hesselgrave 1997).

Kaiser-Permanente, the California-based nonprofit HMO, has invested millions of dollars to build call centers in six of its eight market regions and operates one of the largest call center programs in the nation. In northern California, Kaiser's 2.7 million enrollees generate 20 million calls per year, which are handled by 1,000 customer representatives and registered nurses. Kaiser members use call centers to schedule appointments, refill prescriptions, have health needs triaged, and receive health advice. Nurse advisors manage thousands of Kaiser's chronically ill patients with conditions such as hypertension, diabetes, lung disease, and cancer, utilizing highly evolved patient management protocols. Kaiser is now integrating its call center program with the health plan's interactive web site, Kaiser Permanente Online. Started as a pilot project in 1996 with 1,000 members, Kaiser's web site now has 324,044 registered users. Kaiser, the largest nonprofit HMO with eight million members in 11 states, estimates that 71 percent of its members have online access (*Wall Street Journal* 2001).

SAVINGS ON DEMAND

Call centers that provide consumer health information and referral services can produce significant savings. A recent cost-benefit analysis by a managed care organization has shown $4.75 in savings for every $1.00 invested (Barr, Laufenberg, and Stieckman 1998). Demand management keeps consumers with urgent care needs out of emergency departments by channeling consumers to doctors' offices and other lower-cost health settings. Call centers managed by organizations such as the National Health Enhancement Systems (NHES) have demonstrated savings to health plans and HMOS. NHES's experience is that 60 percent of after-hours calls are for pediatric care. The majority of these calls can be managed by telephone triage and self-management or referred for a next-day physician office visit (Hesselgrave 1997).

The growing emphasis on demand management, disease management, and care coordination is in conflict with the historic role of call centers in creating demand through information and referral services. Some busy call centers, such as the one operated by Sarasota Memorial Hospital in Florida, have split the consumer information and referral function from care management. Routine consumer calls are managed by non-RNS, whereas more complex patient inquiries will be given nurse triage and counseling. Consumers choose from two toll-free telephone numbers to help channel calls to the most appropriate call center.

Integrated delivery systems may operate more complex call centers, which recognize the joint marketing and care management roles and provide an array of services to meet various consumer needs. In Portland, Oregon, an advanced managed care market, the Providence Health System, migrated from a traditional marketing-oriented call center to an integrated delivery system model based on managing care and costs (Odermann, Petras, and Cook 1998). The Sisters of Providence owns one of the largest HMOS in Oregon and has capitated contracts with other health plans. The health system now offers four distinct services to the organization's health plan members, including:

- the Providence RN line for medical triage and advice;
- the Providence audio library, covering more than 1,000 health topics;
- the Providence resource line for information and referral; and

- the care management line for care coordination and skilled nursing facility placement.

MERGER OF COMMUNICATIONS AND COMPUTER TECHNOLOGIES

Advanced technologies are integrating the functions of communications, information systems, and computer-based networks across America's healthcare systems. According to a recent survey of chief information officers by the College of Healthcare Information Management (CHIM), 73 percent of CIOS have management responsibility for telecommunications (Straub 1998). Initial applications by providers often focus on cost saving and staffing reductions using telecommunications technologies; emphasis is now shifting to improving access and patient satisfaction.

Interactive voice response (IVR) systems are an example of the rapidly growing integration of computers, expert systems, and telecommunications. IVR systems enable callers to access information and direct their calls to the appropriate location without operator assistance. In 1997, the IVR market was an estimated $1.1 billion, according to Cahners In-Stat Group, a high-technology market research firm based in Newton, Massachusetts (Straub 1998).

Call routing and phone mail are frequent applications of IVR, but other uses are growing (Straub 1998).

Health Information Library

Specific information on health conditions is only a telephone call away. HBOC, a health information systems company based in Atlanta, offers a computer-based health information library in which more than 1,000 medical topics can be accessed through an IVR system. Callers to a toll-free number identify their health interests and listen to information on a variety of medical conditions. Consumers can also access a nurse to get personal health information before or after accessing the health information library.

Patient Reminder Calls

Automated patient reminder calls are provided by systems such as ReminderPro, offered by JulySoft, based in Tucson, Arizona. With the automated system, clerical staff can load a digital appointment list with patient names and phone numbers in about five minutes. In Nogales, Arizona, the Mariposa Community Health Center has used the ReminderPro system to substantially reduce its 50 percent no-show rate for scheduled appointments. Calls can be made in both English and Spanish for the center's multilingual patients. The system also calls patients who missed appointments, and patients can reschedule a new appointment using a telephone key pad.

Prescription Refills

Health plans and integrated health systems are employing IVR systems to automate prescription refills. In Seattle, the Group Health Cooperative of Puget Sound handles a daily volume of 10,000 calls for patient appointments and 2,000 calls for customer service. Group Health enrollees who already have a prescription can call into the system, enter the prescription number, and receive the prescription from a consumer-selected choice of Group Health sites. The automated system determines if each request is eligible for a refill and places orders. Currently, Group Health's IVR system is handling 3,000 pharmaceutical refills per hour.

The future of call centers is converging with web sites and the Internet, and the voice-enabled web site is the new killer application. Call centers provide the interactivity that web sites lack. Merging call centers with the Internet enables consumers who enter through a Web portal to ask questions, make appointments, or complete transactions. Some hospital web sites are like beautifully stocked—but totally unstaffed—showrooms. Jupiter Communications reports that 90 percent of all online customers prefer human interactions while they are online, particularly when they are making a selection, a decision, or a purchase (Divis 2001). According to Forrester Research, more than 75 percent of all electronic shopping carts are abandoned before the completion of the sale because of a lack of information or because the transaction is too complicated to complete without some assistance. Experts predict that all web sites will soon integrate voice and data into one application.

MARKETING AND CUSTOMER SERVICE

Call centers are high-visibility, low-cost mechanisms for marketing and customer service. Chicago's Advocate Health Care operates a mega–call center that supports eight hospitals, 3,800 affiliated physicians, and 180 sites of care. Advocate's call center manager, Judith Brown, states, "everything is marketing, from greeters to nurses, to the way we handle the bill. The call center is an integral part of our marketing effort" (Appleby 1998, p. 59). The Advocate system's goal is to be the market leader in service, and the call center is a critical piece of this service strategy. At Advocate, the call center's three RNs and 12 support staff handled 184,000 telephone calls in 1999. The center acts as a central marketing database, handling both inbound phone calls and outbound communications, such as appointment confirmations and direct-to-consumer mailings.

In New York's Mt. Sinai Medical Center, one of the city's largest and busiest hospitals, the Teloquent Distributed Call Center provides support for Mt. Sinai's Doctor Referral and Health Resource Service (Straub 1998). This call center operates five days per week, is staffed by RNs, and handles 2,000 calls each month. Since implementing the Teloquent service, calls are up 55 percent. Patients are directly linked to physician offices with three-way conference calls to schedule appointments, coordinate care, and ensure continuity.

CALL CENTERS BECOME EMERGENCY HOT LINES

Hospital- and health system–based call centers can become emergency hot lines in time of community crisis. In Maine, a huge ice storm paralyzed much of the state in January 1998. The Eastern Maine Medical

Center rapidly converted its distributed call center with only an hour's notice into an emergency hot line. The Medical Center serves a regional population of 100,000 in eastern and central Maine. Many Maine residents live in small towns clustered along the Atlantic coast, and access to medical care is an issue. To improve access and coordinate care, the hospital invested $50,000 in June 1997 to establish the call center 18 months before the massive ice storm hit.

Positive results generated from the call center's emergency medical hot line included the following:

- Medical shelter—The center coordinated the transfer of 41 people, ranging in age from 1 to 88, to new sites for medical shelter.
- Consumer information—In the ten days following the ice storm, the hot line service handled 1,200 additional calls for medical information and medical shelter.
- Productivity—Automated call distribution and triage software enabled the call center to reduce caller bottlenecks and ensured that calls were answered promptly.
- Revenues safeguard—The hot line facilitated access to care at the Medical Center, avoiding the potential lost revenues that could have resulted during the disaster.
- Community service—Despite one of the worst natural disasters ever to hit this region, the Eastern Maine Medical Center was able to fill an immediate need by providing this community service through its call center.

PREVENTIVE MEDICINE

Call centers in the future may spend more time on managing chronically ill consumers, and less on triaging urgent care demands. America's 79 million baby boomers will soon be reaching the stage of their life cycle when chronic illness will become much more common. The shift of focus to chronic illness brings to bear a "predict and manage" paradigm for future call centers that will focus on the 10 to 20 percent of the population who will have chronic health problems and limiting disability conditions and are at higher risk for acute medical events. Kaiser Permanente Foundation Health Plan doubled the number of annual mammograms provided to its members in a pilot program in Texas, where call centers routinely offered to schedule a mammogram for all women callers older than 40 years (Christopherson 1998). No-show rates for mammograms were cut by 75 percent with reminders from the call center.

In Indianapolis, the Summex Corporation is developing integrated healthcare management strategies, which begin with a health risk assessment (HRA) for health plan enrollees and consumers obtaining a comprehensive health appraisal (Hesselgrave 1997). Summex's three-page "Health Monitor" is a self-guided questionnaire that asks consumers to select the most appropriate answers from 64 health-related questions. Each individual receives a personal health risk assessment and specific advice on developing a personal health improvement program. Employers and health plans are given reports that aggregate the health risk information on their employees and enrollees. These aggregates identify clusters of risk areas that could become high-cost factors.

MASS-CUSTOMIZED CARE

Triggered by telephone calls or Internet inquiries, call centers can respond in real time with 24×7 availability. Call centers are a high-tech tool for what marketers call mass customization—giving all customers exactly what they want in an individualized manner. In well-designed call centers, the technology is invisible to patients, who simply want highly responsive, personalized health advice or referrals with minimum waiting time.

The vision of the call center is to provide "one-stop shopping" for the healthcare consumer, according to Brent Ballard, Sarasota Memorial Hospital (Ballard 1998, p. 54). With a single telephone call, healthcare consumers can have their health needs diagosed, be given health advice, schedule an appointment, refill a prescription, and obtain health information—all without leaving their living room. Healthcare call centers harness an array of high-tech telecommunications, computer, and expert systems technologies. But "high-touch" service is as important as "high-tech" efficiency. Call centers are designed for high-touch service to support patient-centered processes, which promote care coordination and are seamless to customers.

Consumer demand for alternative medicine is another driving force in the substitution of technology for scarce practitioners. Call centers may become the trusted source of information on alternative medicine and health promotion, providing online health information, advice, and counseling from a credible source that the community trusts. More than 50 percent of health-oriented web sites today are operated by sources that are not connected to health plans or licensed healthcare providers. Call centers can reliably refer callers or route online inquiries to reputable consumer health web sites such as drkoop.com and mayo.com.

CALL CENTER COSTS AND COMPONENTS

Costs for building and operating call centers can range from $250,000 to $1 million per year, and more. Technology is the cheapest part of the investment, amounting to only 10 percent of the overall cost of operating a center (see Figure 8.2). Call distribution systems can be purchased for about $3,500 per seat, and IVR systems cost $1,500 per telephone port. Computer-telephony integration (CTI) systems begin at $100,000 and can cost more than $1 million for a large call center. Workforce management software costs can range from $50,000 to $80,000. Communications transmission costs will average 25 percent of the five-year budget, whereas staffing is the largest expense, comprising 65 percent of total costs (Durr 1998).

The soaring popularity of call centers harnesses the power of automation, computers, expert systems, telecommunications, and the Internet to increase efficiency in managing the health needs, and costs, of millions of healthcare consumers. Core technology components of call centers typically include several elements (Durr 1998; Barr, Laufenberg, and Stiekman 1998).

Figure 8.2: Five-Year Call Center Cost Elements

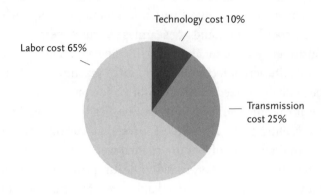

Technology cost 10%

Labor cost 65%

Transmission cost 25%

Source: Durr (1998, p. 13).

Automated Call Distributor

The first line of response when the telephone rings in a call center is the automated call distributor (ACD). The ACD routes calls based on programmed instructions while providing a welcome recording or triggering an IVR application (see below). ACDs distribute the workload among multiple responders in a call center and provide a greeting and instructions if callers are put on hold.

Interactive Voice Response

When calls are received, IVR systems allow callers to select from a number of routing options, including waiting for operator or nurse advisor assistance. Options may include patient identifying information, electronic directory, insurance coverage, appointment scheduling, immediate triage and health advice, and referral. Callers may also obtain information via print, recorded audio, or Internet options.

Graphical User Interface

Newer IVR systems include graphical user interface (GUI) screen application programs that allow call responders to more quickly see and handle information and use the point-and-click technology to route callers. The result is reduced waiting, lower rates of call abandonment, shorter calls, higher staff productivity, and improved patient satisfaction. IVR and GUI systems allow nurses to spend time on more complex inquiries by handling routine calls quickly and electronically.

Computer Telephony Integration

Patient access and care coordination are facilitated by computer-telephony integration. CTI systems use patient indentification information to retrieve patient records from the host system database and display it on screen during the call. Using network screen transfer and predictive dialing (see below), patient records can be electronically routed across the healthcare provider network from the call center to the doctor's office, emergency department, or another care setting.

Predictive Dialers

Outbound calls from the call centers can be electronically programmed to connect with telephones, pagers, or voice mail systems. Predictive dialers can increase staff efficiency by adjusting the sequence of outbound calls to chronically ill patients with the schedules of nurse care managers. Various messages can be electronically delivered, such as appointment or medication reminders.

Telemedicine

As costs are lowered for mini–digital video cameras, the feasibility of universal telemedicine is rapidly arriving and is likely to become reimbursable within the next five years by Medicare and commercial health plans. Video image transmissions over conventional copper twisted-wire cables are slow, but newer asymmetrical digital subscriber lines (ADSLS) can handle substantially higher transmission speeds. Higher bandwith integrated services delivery network lines are now available as a consumer option in many metropolitan areas, running at higher rates of up to 56 kilobytes per second (Kbps). Face-to-face contact via one- or two-way video enhances diagnosis and monitoring by nurses and physicians and is a low-cost way for caregivers to see their patients. Color video images will certainly be preferred in future systems for monitoring chronically ill or high-risk patients. Remote consultation using telemedicine is sure to increase when technology becomes cheaper and more widespread and reimbursement is approved.

Expert Systems

Applications of artificial intelligence in medicine will become widespread as the twenty-first century continues. Disease management companies are already running successful call center programs, which monitor chronically ill patients who are at risk for requiring high-cost healthcare. Predictive dialers call patients, who are queried on their health status by IVR systems. Patient responses are quickly analyzed against preset parameters before the nurse or physician even gets on the telephone line with the patient. The system flags any clinical indicators, pulls up recent data, and can even generate preliminary diagnosis and treatment information according to preprogrammed algorithms.

Telemetry

Automated diagnostic devices can record and transmit patient information electronically, further speeding the monitoring of chronically ill patients or managed care enrollees. Devices such as blood pressure cuffs, spirometers, and otoscopes can be attached to a video or data feed source. Data transmission can be digital if the diagnostic devices are linked to a home computer with an RS232 port, and the data can be immediately incorporated into the patient's electronic medical record.

Web Sites and the Internet

Call centers can support and complement web sites operated by providers and health plans and can refer patients to the vast library of Web-based information on service access, medical conditions, and health education, as well as to specific information sources on the web sites of their provider or health plan sponsors. Web users can generate on-line questions, such as how to determine health plan coverage for a desired service, which can be answered in real time or within 24 hours. Consumers seeking information on urgent care conditions can be automatically referred into a live telephone inquiry for nurse triage and real-time information.

Workforce Management Software

Call centers can employ workforce management software to forecast, plan, and schedule staffing. About 25 percent of call centers are currently using workforce management software to organize historical data on call demands (Durr 1998). The software is capable of producing call volume forecasts with remarkable precision, predicting call arrivals by time, day, date, and month. Staffing and scheduling automatically incorporates variables such as shift length, duration of employee breaks, training programs, sick time, and other employee needs and issues.

HIGH TOUCH IS THE "PEOPLE FACTOR"

Although the emphasis in call centers is applied telecommunications and computer technology, the long-term success of call centers will ultimately be based on the high-touch attitudes and service of its staff. The people, not the technology, are the heart of the call center concept. Call center staff are not interchangeable units, especially in healthcare, so consultants advise health plans and providers to take steps to hire and retain committed staffers. Call center work is repetitive, and many centers experience high staff turnover and burnout.

Becoming a staff-centered call center can keep morale high and turnover low by (Nussbaum and Ault 1998):

- hiring people with a service attitude;
- giving call agents constant feedback;
- continuously training call center employees;
- being innovative in breaking up the routine of handling calls;
- measuring productivity and providing incentives;
- displaying real-time data on screen for call agents;
- monitoring calls as a quality control measure;
- creating an ergonomic work environment;
- reducing noise levels; and
- providing call agents with flexible scheduling.

As virtual call centers become more widely adopted, staff can work from a variety of locations, including their home or regional centers, or be distributed among the health plan's or provider systems' multiple settings. Call center technology offers many options for staff deployment, from centralized to decentralized arrays, large to small offices, and single to multiple enterprises. Outsourcing offers further flexibility by using the external firm to provide backup capacity, peak-time backup, and off-hours coverage.

LOOKING FORWARD: CALL CENTERS ARE VIRTUAL MEDICINE

Medicine's virtual-practice era is rapidly arriving. Imagine primary care providers and specialists only seeing patients in their offices when absolutely necessary, with nurse and patient monitoring being conducted the rest of the time from the "electronic physician office," the call center (Barr, Laufenberg, and Stieckman 1998). The technology for this vision of virtual medicine is available now. Physicians and nurses can diagnose conditions, dispense health advice and prescriptions, and monitor patients' outcomes without ever physically touching the patient. The concept of virtual medicine using telecommunications and computer-assisted protocols is now feasible, as well as being merely technologically possible. While regulators bicker over cross-state licensing issues, Internet connectivity is rapidly making the debate academic. Rapid innovation in telecommunications will offer even more modalities for connecting and coordinating care.

In the practice of virtual medicine, doctors and nurses will employ expert systems, cellular telephone and wireless communications, in-home diagnostic centers, remotely directed drug delivery devices and implants, electronic medical records, and personalized web sites for patients. These services can be provided by local health plans or providers or from remotely located call centers that provide the full range of information and demand management services under an outsourcing arrangement. Or providers can develop a shared call center, such as the Southwest Florida Regional Call Center initiated by Sarasota Memorial Hospital on Florida's west coast, which makes cost-effective use of its technology investment by operating 24 hours per day, seven days per week in partnership with local hospitals (Ballard 1998).

Call centers will become *care centers* in the new millennium. The aging of the population is the obvious challenge for employers, managed care organizations, and government. As the baby boom generation reaches age 50 and beyond, health expenditures will experience a sustained demographic upward push for the next 30 years. Today's $1.3 trillion healthcare economy consumes 14 percent of America's gross domestic product, but the federal Commerce Department has predicted that health expenditures could almost double in ten years to more than $2 trillion. Internet-enabled, guideline-supported, and customer-centered call centers are very promising as a better, faster, cheaper solution for America's health needs in the twenty-first century.

STRATEGIC IMPLICATIONS

The patient is the last frontier of health cost management. If health costs are to be maintained at sustainable levels despite a rapidly aging population, consumers must take more responsibility for maintaining their health and making more efficient use of the health system. Call centers are a promising new strategy that can link patients with providers in a way that is more convenient, lowers costs, and is immediately responsive to consumer demands.

Seeing More Patients with Fewer Staff. Better, faster, cheaper processes are needed for diagnosing, treating, and monitoring millions of Americans who will have chronic illnesses. Studies show that 40 to 80 percent of all patients entering the health system do not need a physician (Barr, Laufenberg, and Stiekman 1998). Call centers could become the centerpieces of innovative care management processes, which substitute technology for scarce labor. They could also help solve healthcare's looming labor shortages at a time when baby boom-age doctors and nurses are likely to retire just as the "age wave" crests.

Empowering Technologies. Call centers are the leading edge of a new wave of empowering technologies that can facilitate America's 275 million health consumers to take more responsibility for their own health. Telecommunications and virtual medicine can overcome traditional barriers to access, such as insurance coverage, distance, transportation, and limited information.

Self-Health Is Cost-Effective Medicine. The combination of universal Internet access, cheap telecommunications, customized health information, and nurse-supplied health advice can be a powerful strategy for the coming era of self-health. Integrated health systems and health plans must become information suppliers and communications enablers. Large numbers of consumers will employ call centers and other empowering technologies to promote their optimum health.

REFERENCES

American Productivity and Quality Center (APQC). 1998. "Best Practices for World Class Call Centers." *Healthcare Benchmarks*, pp. 164–65. Houston, TX: APQC.

Appleby, C. 1998. "Dialing." *Hospitals & Health Networks* 73 (10): 58–60.

Ballard, B. 1998. "The Evolution of a Call Center at Sarasota Memorial Hospital." *Health Management Technology* 19 (10): 54–56.

Barr, J. L., S. Laufenberg, and B. L. Stieckman. 1998. "Creating a Vision for Your Call Center." *Healthcare Information Management* 12 (2): 71–85.

Chin, T. L. 1998. "Call Centers Improve Service, Carry Out Managed Care Goals." *Health Data Management* February: 122–27.

Christopherson, K. A. 1998. "Call Centers in Healthcare: The Experience of One Health Maintenance Organization." *Healthcare Information Management* 12 (2): 53–55.

Divis, K. 2001. "Customer Needs Can Be Better Met by 'Voice'." COR *Healthcare Market Strategist* 2 (2): 1, 16–18.

Durr, W. 1998. "A Call Center Primer." *Healthcare Information Management* 12 (2): 5–17.

Frost & Sullivan. 1999. "Increasingly Competitive Call Center Market Is Prompting Market Participants to Rise to the Challenge," [Online press release.] January 26, pp. 1–3. Mountain View, CA: Frost & Sullivan.

Hesselgrave, B. 1997. "Dialing for Diagnosis." *InfoCARE* July/August: 57–64.

Krup, L. B. 1999. "Call Center Trends," January 26. [Online press release.] Philadelphia: CenterCore.

Millenson, M. 1999. *Demand Medical Excellence: Doctors and Accountability in the Information Age.* Chicago: University of Chicago Press.

Nussbaum, G. M., and S. P. Ault. 1998. "One Ringy Dingy: Call Centers of the Nineties." *Healthcare Information Management* 12 (2): 107–18.

Odermann, M., G. J. Petras, and J. Cook. 1998. "Providence Health Plan Call Center: A Case Study in Innovation and Integration." *Healthcare Information Management* 12 (2): 121–26.

Serb, C. 1998. "A Con Job." *Hospitals & Health Networks* 72 (8): 58–59.

Straub, H. 1998. "Lives and Livelihoods on the Line." *Health Management Technology* 19 (10): 24–30.

Wall Street Journal. 2001. "'Information Therapy' May Help Treat Patients." [Online news brief.] News Briefs, February 2, p. 2. Southfield, MI: Superior Consultant.

CHAPTER NINE

Telemedicine: A New Foundation for Healthcare Delivery

KEY CONCEPTS: *Telemedicine • Telehealth • Bandwith • Virtual reality • Telepresence •* PCS *•* PDA *• Plug and play •* VPN

INTRODUCTION: Telemedicine is becoming the foundation of a whole new way to deliver healthcare, both in the United States and internationally. Telemedicine's growth is one of the most exciting examples of technology's ability to transform and improve a key industry. Visionary clinicians and entrepreneurs are harnessing the transformational power of the Internet, telecommunications, and information technology to solve many of healthcare's most vexing problems. Early experiments with telemedicine were limited by the high costs and limited flexibility of interactive video, but recently, the focus of telemedicine has shifted to the Internet. Costs for telemedicine systems are falling rapidly, and digital video technology is providing small, low-cost cameras for two-way Web-enabled telecommunication with real-time streaming video. At the beginning of the twenty-first century, telemedicine is poised to become a widespread and cost-effective tool for improving the delivery of healthcare.

"**tele•med•i•cine** n: the combined use of telecommunications and computer technologies to improve the efficiency and effectiveness of health care service, also a liberating caregivers from traditional constraints of space and time; **b** empowering consumers to make informed choices in a competitive marketplace

—*Jeffrey C. Bauer and Marc A. Ringel (1999)*

Telemedicine is beginning to restructure and redefine healthcare delivery systems around the globe. Many traditional concepts of health and medicine will be reassessed in the process. The concept of telemedicine appeared on the fringes of American medicine in the 1960s. Linking patients and providers remotely became possible when telecommunications systems developed the capacity for transmitting interactive video, and a revolution in medical practice started when telecommunications and computers converged during the last decade of the twentieth century. What began as a few experiments to link remote sites in the same state via video has become a fast-growing number of applications that use a variety of technologies to transcend traditional barriers of place and time.

Telemedicine's potential reach is now truly global, bringing healthcare even to the summit of Mt. Everest. In 1996, a party of climbers stranded high on that mountain was able to link with medical advisors using a wireless Internet connection and low-earth orbit satellite telecommunications. A team of vendors and academics, including AT&T, Logical Design Solutions, Massachusetts Institute of Technology, and Yale University, organized the Everest Extreme Expedition (E3) program to monitor climbers in the brutal conditions of high altitudes (Bauer and Ringel 1999). The system they designed collected data from physiologic sensors and digital video cameras carried by mountaineers, transmitting down to a base camp equipped with a miniaturized intensive care unit, complete with a portable three-dimensional (3-D) ultrasound. From base camp, data were relayed to the INMARSAT satellite hovering over the Indian Ocean and rebroadcast to Malaysia, which speeded it by ISDN links from California to experts at Yale and the Walter Reed Army Hospital. One team member, Dr. Beck Wethers, a Texas pathologist, was brought back to life after spending a night exposed on the mountain. Although E3 could not prevent the tragic deaths of several MT. Everest climbers, it is a remarkable demonstration of the state-of-the-practice technology now available to support telemedicine in new and different ways.

A BRIEF HISTORY OF TELEMEDICINE

Doctors and their patients have longed for a technology solution to the problem of remote access to medical care. Three projects are recognized as the earliest examples of applications that ultimately evolved to become modern telemedicine (Preston 1999, pp. 4–6):

- University of Nebraska—In 1959, psychiatrists at the University of Nebraska School of Medicine began using a microwave video link to consult with patients and health professionals at a state mental hospital located more than 100 miles away.
- NASA—The National Aeronautics and Space Administration (NASA) established a medical communications system with an Indian reservation in Arizona in the early 1960s for developing capabilities to provide healthcare over large distances.
- Mass General—A group of doctors at Massachusetts General Hospital began using a video network in 1968 to examine emergency patients at Logan Airport because traffic jams often prevented travel via the connecting tunnel under Boston Harbor.

Based on the success of these early projects, interactive video linkages between rural and urban health systems became relatively common by the 1980s. Without traveling to the city, patients in remote communities could be examined by specialists at large urban medical centers. Rural health professionals could use the same equipment for continuing education programs or administrative meetings with distant colleagues. Interactive video provided an unprecedented alternative to getting the patient and the doctor together for a medical visit.

Of course, the parties to a virtual encounter still had to "meet" at the same time, if not in the same place (Kvedar, Menn, and Loughlin 1998). Scheduling constraints could still be inconvenient or expensive for busy doctors. They often had to choose between interrupting in-office appointments or keeping online patients waiting while line charges continued to mount. And costs were prohibitively expensive, averaging more than $1,000 per telemedicine visit after factoring in the investment in satellite telecommunications equipment.

First-generation telemedicine eliminated one significant barrier to access, place, but it often cost more time and money than traditional face-to-face care. Insurers' initial resistance to paying for telemedicine consultations was understandable. Interactive video created new possibilities for doctor-patient interaction, but the changes were not dramatic enough to shake the foundations of healthcare.

Second-generation telemedicine was launched in the mid-1990s with a variety of new platform-crossing applications that also overcame the barrier of time. In dermatology, digitized photographs of skin lesions could be taken at the patient's convenience and sent via the Internet to a dermatologist for review at a later time (Murphy et al. 1972). The web site of the Internet Dermatology Society at http://www .telemedicine.org shows actual examples of electronic images that are shared between dermatologists and other doctors. In radiology, computerized tomographs (CT) and magnetic resonance image (MRI) scans could be used to create three-dimensional images for downloading to geographically dispersed specialists who share interpretations and research cases or even plan surgical interventions. In its second generation, high-speed telecommunications gave telemedicine more speed and bandwith. However, it did not overcome the cost issues, and access was still limited.

More recently, the focus of telemedicine has shifted to the Internet. Web-based telemedicine applications promise lower costs, almost universal access, and multimodal capability to transmit a variety of data and images. In home care, chronically ill patients are now using new devices to analyze vital signs and body fluids and sending the results to their doctor's office and to their online medical record for ongoing monitoring. Medicine can now follow the patient almost anywhere. For an introduction to these new and emerging applications in surgery, see the Wiley Interscience web site at http://www.interscience.wiley.com /cas/ and follow links to specific areas of interest. Also visit the Virtual Human Gallery at http://www.gsm.com to view thumbnail sketches of sample 3-D images constructed from real tissue, or http://www.ai.mit .edu/projects/medical-vision/ to see noninvasively generated 3-D images that can easily be shared over the Internet.

As exciting as these second- and third-generation innovations may be, telemedicine has not attained the status of a mature product. The Mayo Clinic specialists in Rochester, Minnesota, routinely teleconsult with their colleagues in Arizona and Florida, and Temple, Texas–based Scott and White Clinic has 16 satellite telelinked clinics, but these examples are still early models. The telemedicine revolution has just begun. Telemedicine is now being envisioned as a solution to a wider array of problems, such as reaching out to the medically underserved in urban areas. In Los Angeles, the Charles R. Drew University of Medicine recently opened its third urban telemedicine site, this one providing pediatric care (Tieman 2001); Drew's first two clinics provide eye care in public housing projects. The telemedicine network is being underwritten by a federal grant from the Department of Health and Human Services and a foundation gift from the California Telehealth and Telemedicine Center in Sacramento, plus a $2 million development grant from Los Angeles County.

TELEMEDICINE BY ANY OTHER NAME ...

The telemedicine revolution in medical care has taken off without a leader. The origin of the term telemedicine is usually credited to the physician group mentioned at the beginning of this chapter, who created a video link between Massachusetts General Hospital and Logan Airport in Boston (Murphy et al. 1972). But no identifiable person, company, or government agency can claim ownership or control of this emerging movement, a situation which has allowed several different designations to be attached to this new way of delivering healthcare. Network medicine, telehealth, digital medicine, distributed healthcare, and a few other names can be found in current use.

The semantic difference is intended in some cases to make a point. "Telehealth," the most common alternative term to describe telemedicine, is used intentionally to differentiate healthcare from medical care—that is, to draw a distinction between a comprehensive (holistic) view and the more focused model of medical doctors. The differences between health and medicine are worth discussing, but they should not obscure the real issue. The distinction between telemedicine and telehealth is not really meaningful. Whatever the label, the convergence of telecommunications and computers will change the future for everyone, from new age healer to medical subspecialist. This use of telemedicine in this book reflects the most common practice and implies no disrespect for alternate terms.

TELEMEDICINE AND E-COMMERCE: COMPLETING THE DIGITAL TRANSFORMATION

Information systems and networked computers have existed in the health field for more than two decades, but early applications focused on computer time sharing, group purchasing, and electronic claims. Clinical applications were slower to follow because of cost constraints and limited access to telecommunications technology by providers. The broader realm of e-commerce in healthcare began to attract a lot of attention in the late 1990s, as commercialization of the World Wide Web began in earnest. Hospitals, insurance companies, pharmaceutical manufacturers, retail drug stores, and other providers of medical services are now all migrating their products and services to the Web. E-commerce in healthcare, often called "e-health," is opening new market opportunities for suppliers and customers in the medical care industry, including:

- connections—selling communications linkages, including everything from public Internet access through Internet service providers (ISPS) to extranets and virtual private networks (VPNS) (visit www.v-one.com to consult a collection of white papers on network security services being used in healthcare);
- applications—offering access to the latest clinical or managerial software on an as-needed basis, effectively transforming the software business from site-licensed sales of floppy disks or CD-ROMS to online rentals with charges based on volume;

- products—creating virtual shopping centers that sell everything from prescription drugs and sundries to a complete range of supplies for hospitals and other delivery organizations;
- services—providing clinical consultations, real-time analysis of medical data, remote "telepresence" surgery, patient monitoring, and other twenty-first-century versions of care previously delivered in the traditional doctor-patient relationship; and
- information—offering the use of specific databases, electronic libraries, and other knowledge resources to inform the actions of buyers and sellers in the medical marketplace. Well-established examples of such online services include onhealth.com, drkoop.com, emedicine.com, mayohealth.com, WebMD.com, cdc.gov/nchs, and intellihealth.com.

With the development of these new business relationships, the distinction between telemedicine and e-health is blurring rapidly. More fundamentally, the convergence of these trends is part of the digital transformation of healthcare. Creative and visionary business leaders, provider organizations, and health plans will find growing opportunities in one or more of these market areas. Whether the new market is characterized as telemedicine or e-health is inconsequential. Semantic nuances should not divert attention from the skyrocketing number of ways in which networked computers are revolutionizing the delivery of healthcare.

CHANGES IN THE PRACTICE OF TELEMEDICINE

In the early days—before 1997 or so—most telemedicine interactions required a refrigerator-sized console full of electronic equipment or a dedicated suite, essentially a mini–television studio, at each end of the clinical encounter. All participants, from the remotely based specialist at one end to the patient and referring physician at the other, had to be in their places at the appointed time. A small team of computer and video technicians was necessary at both sites as well. The process may have seemed magical from some perspectives, but it was also cumbersome, expensive, and time consuming compared with a traditional doctor-patient visit.

Today, the basic equipment of telemedicine is miniaturized, portable, and relatively inexpensive. A complete home telemedicine kit, including a video camera and digital monitors for vital signs and body fluids, can fit on the top of a small table and be plugged into a regular telephone outlet. Visit http://www.americantelecare.com and http://www.americanmeddev.com to see examples of modern homecare kits for telemedicine. The typical unit at the receiving end in a doctor's office or hospital is not much larger or more costly. This technology is evolving very rapidly. The next generation of telemedicine equipment will likely include devices that hook up directly to the home cable television system.

Information appliances, small devices with built-in computer chips and Internet connections, will also help reshape the future of telemedicine. A patient with serious respiratory or cardiac problems may wear clothing imbedded with lightweight biosensors that record critical information and send it periodically to the patient's care manager and online medical record. These devices will alert patient and caregiver when the data suggest an impending crisis. Not long ago, doctors grimly joked that the first sign of a myocardial infarction was death. Soon, it will be the information appliance's verbal command telling the patient to head immediately to the nearest emergency room—along with instructions, generated by a built-in GPS, on how to get there.

Wireless technologies are further expanding the potential of telemedicine. A considerable amount of medical information will be exchanged over next-generation wireless telephones, called personal communications systems (PCSs), linked to the Internet and local infrared or radio wave networks. Personal digital assistants are already linking health professionals to medical records and health plan databases. The convergence of PCS and PDA devices will allow physicians, nurses, pharmacists, and other health professionals to review data provided by patients from their homes, make diagnoses, and order prescriptions whenever and wherever they may.

PHYSICIAN REIMBURSEMENT: THE FINAL BARRIER TO TELEMEDICINE

Is telemedicine an idea whose time has come, or just a blip on the cyber-screen to which few physicians will respond? The answer depends on whether and when doctors will get paid for online work (Bauer and Coile 2000). The question of paying physicians for online practice may have seemed academic as recently as three years ago. Telemedicine was synonymous with interactive video consultations between rural patients and urban specialists, financed by federal grants to cover its high costs. A survey by Medem, an e-health network sponsored by the American Medical Association, found that only one doctor in ten was currently communicating with patients by e-mail, but that 50 percent of physicians would be interested in doing so if they were reimbursed (Wheat 2001).

Momentum for acceptance of telemedicine by patients, physicians, and payers is now growing. Several trends are accelerating the convergence of telecommunications and computers in medicine:

- The Internet moved from the fringe to the center of healthcare in the final years of the twentieth century, demonstrating its potential to reinvent medicine and healthcare delivery.
- Consumers began flooding cyberspace, using the services of tens of thousands of Internet-based health information providers.
- The doctor-patient relationship was liberated from long-standing constraints of place and time as telemedicine escaped the shackles of real-time video and entered the flexible world of store-and-forward technology.
- Membership in the American Telemedicine Association more than doubled between 1998 and 2000, as did the number of vendors demonstrating their products in telemedicine trade shows.
- E-health was discovered by practitioners, attracting thousands of health administrators and clinicians to major conferences that

showed how the Internet could enhance almost every economic relationship in the industry.

- Payment is becoming available, as a few Internet-savvy health plans have begun paying doctors for telemedicine visits with patients (Galdabini 2000).

Many barriers—not the least of which is physicians' traditional reluctance to change—stand in the way of establishing telemedicine on a scale that would compel insurers to pay for it routinely. Insurers have not yet accepted a common definition of a "tele-visit." However, data suggest that consumers are leading the way, and physicians are not far behind. Telemedicine's growth is impressive, from a few thousand rural patients getting video consultations with urban specialists to tens of millions of Americans using the Internet for healthcare in fewer than five years. Political support for telemedicine is also growing; relaxation of Medicare restrictions on payment for telemedicine is a strong possibility in the near future.

Recent developments suggest that health insurers and managed care organizations may be ready to reimburse telemedicine. First Health announced in early 2001 that it would be the first national health benefits company to reimburse physicians for e-visits (Wheat 2001). The company will pay $25 for each e-mail consultation and not charge a consumer copayment. First Health has signed up approximately 15 self-insured companies to participate. The company is starting with chronically ill patients who have existing relationships with physicians. The e-visits will take place using First Health's technology network through a secure web site to prevent unauthorized access. Patient inquiries will be answered over the Web within 48 hours.

THE E-SOLUTION TO AMERICA'S ACCESS CRISIS

Telemedicine and the digital transformation of healthcare could redefine the issue of access. Attention was focused almost entirely on uninsured Americans during the last half of the twentieth century, but concern in the twenty-first century may shift to people who do not use the Internet and the Web. The digital divide is a major concern where

Internet access is the difference between informed healthcare users and those without easy access to online health advice and information. Today, some 100 million Americans have Internet-enabled access to healthcare, but the majority of Americans still cannot connect with their providers online or otherwise participate in the electronic marketplace.

Telemedicine can be the deciding factor in the feasibility of providing health services to remote, thinly populated areas. In Moab, Utah, the 36-bed Allen Memorial Hospital arranged to have data from the patients in the hospital's small intensive care unit wired to St. Mark's Hospital, located 250 miles away in Salt Lake City. St. Mark's is a 306-bed tertiary care hospital specializing in cardiac care (Bauer and Ringel 1999). The interactive network, called SiteLink by VitalCom, the hospitals' telecommunications partner, was established in 1997. During the first five months of operation, real-time remote monitoring was credited for reducing transfers from Allen Memorial's ICU by 82 percent and keeping an extra $80,000 of revenues in the rural facility while saving an equal amount in transfer costs. Surgeons in Moab have been willing to perform higher-risk surgeries, further boosting hospital revenues, because the doctors have confidence that the postoperative care will be monitored from Salt Lake City by some of the best experts in Utah.

Inspiring examples like Allen Memorial demonstrate the feasibility of telemedicine, but they just begin to define this technology's innovative potential to address America's access problems. Telemedicine is no longer just a mechanism for providing virtual consultations to patients in rural areas that cannot afford medical specialists. It is becoming the foundation of a reinvented healthcare system, putting offline people at a disadvantage no matter where they live. Consequently, regulators and legislators may need to re-examine the Telecommunications Act of 1984 and other laws that hinder the provision of affordable telecommunications to all consumers, urban or rural. For example, restrictions on local carriers' abilities to cross local access and transport areas (LATAS) may unnecessarily prevent access to telemedicine services in a variety of geographic areas.

Access solutions via telemedicine may be hindered or advanced by future government policy regarding telecommunications and the

Internet. Deregulation was necessary in the 1980s because the long-standing theory of public utilities was rendered obsolete by advances in technology. Communications technologies such as wireless systems have continued to change in ways that were not envisioned even in the mid-1990s, much less in the mid-1980s. Dynamic policies are needed to reflect the evolutionary reality of twenty-first-century technology and its potential contributions to critical industries like healthcare. Telemedicine will ultimately prevail, but forward-looking access policy would help avoid unnecessary roadblocks along the way.

BANDWIDTH AVAILABILITY FOR TELEMEDICINE

The growth of telemedicine will require a lot of telecommunications capacity, and bandwith is a measure of that capacity. The amount of information that can be sent over a communications channel in one second is called bandwidth. It is analogous to the amount of water that can be pumped through a pipe, such as gallons per second. In digital telecommunications, bandwidth is generally measured in bits per second. A bit is a binary string of eight digits, for example, 01100101. Some telecommunications "pipes" have more bandwidth than others. They are called broadband channels. For example, a fiberoptic cable can carry many more bits of information per second than a regular copper telephone line, known as a "twisted pair." On the other hand, several telephone lines can be linked together to produce comparable bandwidth, such as with T-1 lines. Other common telecommunications pipes include microwave and coaxial cable. With respect to telemedicine, the transmission of clinical images such as x-rays, digital photographs, or video requires a certain amount of bandwidth to be clinically useful. An analogous comparison would be that of a garden hose to a firehose: the more time sensitive the delivery, the bigger the telecommunications pipeline needs to be.

Bandwidth has been one of the major barriers to the growth of telemedicine. In the pioneering days of telemedicine, early adopters used dedicated broadband video networks, which were necessary for live video. Although bandwith capacity is increasing exponentially, it is still not widely installed in doctors' offices, patients' homes, and other locations where telemedicine has potential application. Recent mergers between telephone and cable companies suggest that bandwidth will be abundantly available to the healthcare industry in the near future, and technologies for expanding and creating bandwith are evolving very rapidly. Engineers are continuously discovering new ways to push more data through a given pipe, and multibillion dollar investments are being made to build telecommunications networks.

Bandwidth will not be a major constraint on the growth of telemedicine in the twenty-first century. Competition is rapidly bringing broadband communications to more locations in more geographic areas, and engineers continue to expand the capacity of existing channels. As shown in reports recently issued by the American Telemedicine Association (see Resources at http://www.atmeda.org), these advances suggest that many previous forecasts of the growth in telemedicine most likely understate the economic potential in this market. Infrastructure and capacity are growing much faster than expected.

Users should expect more innovation in creating or expanding bandwith. The commercial stakes are high, and healthcare is not the only customer. Clinically useful video images can now be sent over regular telephone lines because signals can be compressed with software. Compression involves the suppression of detail that does not change from frame to frame, such as still backgrounds, so that only vital information is pumped through the pipe. This new capability dramatically expands the applications of telemedicine in home care, but it was unimaginable as recently as a year or two ago. The growing use of digital diagnostic devices also allows better use of narrowband channels because digitally acquired signals are more efficient than comparable analog signals.

STANDARDS FOR TELECOMMUNICATIONS

The early years of telemedicine were marked by development of some impressive systems to transmit interactive video, diagnostic images, databases, continuing education programs, meetings, and other professional activities. However, deployment was often hindered because different manufacturers' units could not communicate with each other. Many vendors offered "closed" systems using proprietary technology, which forced purchasers to buy identical equipment for each site where telemedicine would be delivered. One rural hospital might have vendor A's system to link local patients with distant specialists and vendor B's equipment to send x-rays for interpretation by urban radiologists. The inefficiency is obvious: the two different systems effectively did the same job but could not work together at either site.

The meteoric rise of the Internet since the mid-1990s is rapidly overcoming the problem of vendor-to-vendor incompatibility due to lack of standards. "Open" systems are the new norm in telemedicine at the beginning of the twenty-first century. For a vendor to be successful today, its equipment should be "IP" enabled, that is, ready to share information with other devices in the standard language of the Internet. The look and feel of Web-transmitted images will be much enhanced by extensible markup language (XML), a widely adopted software that is rapidly becoming the standard for virtual reality images on the Internet (Bosak and Bray 1999). The prevailing concept in electronic data interchange systems has quickly become universal "plug and play." By demanding equipment that operates using standardized electronic interfaces, hospitals, doctors, and other telemedicine users can buy equipment from different vendors and know that everything will work together. For industry news about advances in the compatibility of telemedicine equipment, visit http://www.atsp.org, the web site of the Association of Telemedicine Service Providers.

Scalability, a related concept of considerable importance, is the built-in capability for equipment to grow with needs and change with technology. It allows basic devices to be upgraded via the replacement of more powerful components rather than the purchase of a whole new piece of equipment. The early days of telemedicine were characterized by one-size-fits-all systems, which kept many potential users out of the market because they only needed a fraction of the large-scale capacity built into the available devices. More recently, manufacturers have responded to market demands by building equipment that can be expanded. Cameras, storage units, equipment racks, and other system components can now be upgraded when the expense is justified by increases in volume or improvements in technology.

The growing acceptance of common standards is leading to intense competition in the telemedicine equipment business. The market has shifted dramatically from the closed systems of the 1990s to open platforms in the realm of "commercial, off-the-shelf" (COTS) products and "plain old telephone service" (POTS). The growth of COTS and POTS has also favored international applications of telemedicine, enabling impressive demonstration projects in less-developed countries that lack the infrastructure and resources to support technologically advanced systems. For an overview of innovative work being done in remote geographic areas outside the United States, explore the Projects section of http://www.meditac.com, the web site of the Medical Informatics and Technology Applications Consortium of NASA and the medical campus of Virginia Commonwealth University.

The development of electronic standards has also had a positive effect on healthcare information. Even with compatible hardware, a telemedicine system will be ineffective if all software does not handle information in the same way. A digitized x-ray or medical record received by a consulting specialist would be useless if the file could not be opened simply because the sender created it with incompatible software. This problem is immediately recognizable to anyone who has been unable to open an e-mail attachment. The e-mail text conforms to a universal standard, but in many cases the attached file does not.

Software compatibility through standards has started to receive as much attention as interoperability of hardware. Most teleradiology equipment now conforms to digital image and communications in medicine (DICOM) standards that ensure images are stored and transmitted in a consistent format. After years of discussion and development, a consortium of government agencies, providers, and information technology organizations are defining Health Level–7 (HL-7) as the uniform standard for compatibility of text files such as medical records and billing forms. The communication of medical forms is also being facilitated by the replacement of HTML (hypertext markup language), the protocols that enable collection of information via forms on web pages, with XML, a more flexible interface.

BRINGING DOWN THE COSTS OF TELEMEDICINE

Until recently, the cost of telemedicine systems was a common barrier to entry. Early adopters had to buy far more capacity than they needed and maintain dedicated lines that were seldom used more than a few hours a day. The initial capital investment and high fixed operating costs gave telemedicine a reputation of being very expensive. Only large provider organizations like the Mayo Clinic or government-subsidized rural hospitals could usually afford to enter the world of telemedicine in the 1990s. Today, the future of telemedicine is very different from its past because of fundamental improvements in bandwidth, standards, and affordability. The market potential of telemedicine is about to undergo a tremendous leap forward, as low-cost telecommunications technology makes telehealth much more affordable.

Beginning late in the 1990s, the costs of telemedicine began to fall due to growth in the service provider business. Taking a cue from ISPs that spread the cost of servers and dedicated lines over large numbers of occasional users, this new type of telemedicine vendor invested in high-capacity systems and "rented" its functions on a per-use or subscription basis. Price competition drove telecommunications carriers to sell fractionated portions of broadband lines, for example, one-half of a T-1 line, and some teleradiology systems were priced on a per-click basis. Medical software systems are also becoming available through applications service providers (ASPs) who charge for downloaded software only as it is used.

HUMAN FACTORS

Technology is often criticized for its failure to respect the cultural values and psychological needs of the populations it affects. Telemedicine is potentially vulnerable to such charges because healthcare is one of the most intrinsically human activities, with a heritage of the healing touch that dates back thousands of years. Telemedicine systems need to be developed with careful attention to human concerns. Privacy, for example, is as important in telemedicine as it is in a face-to-face encounter. Patients may respond poorly to telemedicine if they do not have confidence in the privacy of the encounter. Earphones, not loudspeakers, should be used in open settings to ensure that the patient "visit" remains private. Video monitors should be placed in such a way that only the patient and his or her health professional can see them. Research suggests that cameras should be positioned at eye level, and backgrounds behind the caregiver should give the appearance of a professional setting.

Successful planning and installation of telemedicine systems also require careful attention to human factors. Technology needs to be as transparent as possible to the users. The more cumbersome and intrusive a device, the less likely it will be used. The need to use a keyboard can be a deterrent to anyone who does not type or have much computer keyboard experience. Systems with voice recognition and touch screens will become increasingly common. User training is critical. Neither patient nor practitioner will develop favorable long-term impressions of telemedicine if their first encounters are complicated by lack of familiarity with equipment or procedures.

Some commentators have argued that the growth of telemedicine will be limited by a strong public preference for high touch over high tech. Of course, the healing touch will be important to all the people some of the time and some of the people all the time, but telemedicine's skeptics may be taking the concept of touch too literally. AT&T once advertised the telephone's ability to "reach out and touch someone," a power that can be harnessed by telemedicine. Given a choice between impersonalized face-to-face care and patient-sensitive telemedicine, many consumers will prefer the immediacy and depth of medical services delivered over the telephone or Internet. The benefits of telemedicine—particularly greater convenience, lower costs, and integrated records—will appeal to many people. Acceptance will also grow as people use more technology in other aspects of their daily lives. It is hard to remember that the telephone was threatening and unpopular when it was introduced to the general public a century ago.

TEN CHALLENGES IN THE ACCEPTANCE OF TELEMEDICINE

Like any new concept that challenges a well-established way of doing things, telemedicine raises a host of policy, payment, and regulatory issues. Health professionals, consumers, policy analysts, health plans, and elected officials will be grappling with these questions for years to come. The solutions will change with technology and public perception, but discussion is already framed around several key issues.

1. Professional Licensure and Malpractice

The privilege to practice medicine or other health disciplines is controlled by state-granted licenses. Practitioners are only allowed to offer their services in states in which they are licensed, reflecting the legal concept that a patient harmed by professional negligence will have standing to sue in courts of the state in which malpractice was committed. For example, a patient harmed by a doctor in Colorado cannot pursue the doctor in a Nebraska court. But what can a patient in Colorado do if harm resulted from a telemedicine consultation with a doctor practicing and licensed only in Nebraska?

2. Conflicting State Regulations

States are addressing in different ways the regulations issues raised by telemedicine. The status of state regulations affecting telemedicine, including payment as well as licensure, is evolving very rapidly. Consult http://www.legamed.com to review an up-to-date list of each state's rules and regulations on the practice of telemedicine. No national legislation currently exists to regulate interstate telemedicine, and states are taking a variety of approaches, including ignoring the issue. A model state statute has been developed, which nine states have adopted as of 2001. Some states have passed laws that require health professionals to be licensed in the state in which the patient was located at the time of care. Others have granted limited licenses for telemedicine, for example, allowing a doctor from another state to make a limited number of consultations—say, ten per year—across a state boundary. Many experts expect the ultimate resolution to be federal licenses for telemedicine, but the time frame for this possible outcome is unpredictable. Some multistate compacts have already been formed to recognize licenses for purposes of practicing telemedicine, notably in nursing.

3. Internet Pharmacies

The introduction of online pharmacies raises a related issue. Internet drugstores may be staffed by pharmacists licensed in many different states, yet the pharmacies are not licensed in every state. The best way to solve the problem is far from clear, but an answer may be coming from the profession. The National Association of State Boards of Pharmacy has established a uniform set of standards. Virtual drugstores can apply for certification as Verified Internet Pharmacy Practice Sites (VIPPSS) and display the program's logo on their web page. This alternative to state licensure is being closely watched because self-regulation is a cherished goal of most Internet industry insiders.

4. Reimbursement

Telemedicine developed an early reputation for being very expensive, as was true in the days of interactive video. As a result, health insurers and fiscal intermediaries have generally taken a very restrictive approach to paying for care provided over telemedicine networks. Medicare effectively sets the prevailing national standard, paying only for telemedicine when the patient resides in a federally designated health professional shortage area (HPSA). The Balanced Budget Act of 1997 mandated several studies to determine the actual costs of telemedicine, and no major changes in federal policy are expected until the results of these studies are presented in late 2001 or 2002. Unfortunately, the demonstration programs are almost exclusively based on interactive video, so the day-to-day technology and practice of telemedicine will be several generations ahead of the government-financed projects by the time they report their results. Recent enactment of the Benefits Improvement and Protection Act (BIPA) of 2000 has somewhat liberalized the Medicare payment policy for telemedicine.

5. Health Plans

Acceptance of telemedicine by major health plans could jump-start telemedicine's acceptance by physicians and hospitals. Some promising payment policies are being implemented in the private sector. Several health maintenance organizations have been particularly progressive in their use of telemedicine, and some traditional health plans have begun to relax payment restrictions. The key to progress most likely lies in the private sector where insurers can respond relatively quickly to mounting evidence that telemedicine is cost-effective. Consumer demand will also help pay for more telemedicine in the future. Mounting evidence suggests that people are willing to pay out-of-pocket for the convenience of telemedicine, especially for home care services. Finally, the accelerating shift from employer-controlled insurance, for example, defined benefits, to individually directed insurance, such as defined contributions, should promote telemedicine. Many consumers will want telemedicine coverage in their customized health plans.

6. Consumer Acceptance

Telemedicine has yet to meet a broad test of consumer acceptance. Most pilot projects in telemedicine have occurred in rural areas, where patients have limited access options. In these early demonstrations, consumer satisfaction is generally favorable, with studies showing that many patients find both advantages and disadvantages with telemedicine. Advantages for patients seem to outweigh the disadvantages, and overall consumer satisfaction tends to increase with exposure. Because lack of insurance reimbursement is consistently seen as a major disadvantage of telemedicine, consumer acceptance can be expected to increase as health plans cover more telemedicine care.

7. Quality

As a new approach, telemedicine raises understandable concerns about quality. The safety and appropriateness of care delivered via telemedicine have not yet been conclusively demonstrated, but research suggests that telemedicine can be the foundation of very good care. Many unanswered questions remain, due to the relative lack of clinical or outcomes data, but telemedicine is arguably ahead of traditional care in one important dimension of quality—use of practice guidelines. Studies of practice guidelines have consistently identified a positive contribution to clinical outcomes, and telemedicine organizations have been actively involved in developing guidelines that focus attention on quality control in all aspects of patient-provider interactions. For detailed information about clinical guidelines, see the Telemedicine Resources section of http://www.americantelemed .org and link to areas of specific interest. Telemedicine is also more likely than conventional care to be linked to electronic medical record systems that improve clinical decision making and reduce practice errors.

8. Telemedicine on the Web

Telemedicine is rapidly migrating to the Internet, but most of the evaluated demonstrations have focused on two-way satellite television, an expensive and limited media. Today, the Internet offers low-cost access to a wealth of medical information and the potential to link patients on a 24 × 7 basis with doctors, hospitals, and health plans. More than 50 million Americans are now accessing the Web for health information, but healthcare professionals, health plans, and government regulators have concerns about the quality of information on the Internet. Computer communications are not peer reviewed. False or misleading information can pass over the lines just as easily as reports from the most respected medical journals. One of telemedicine's greatest challenges is to develop user-friendly tools that help consumers separate good information from bad.

9. Cost

Telemedicine is rapidly becoming less expensive, which is not surprising, as the costs of its basic components—computers, telecommunications, and digital devices—are falling fast. Cost reductions are reinforced as telemedicine expands beyond interactive video to encompass many lower-cost technologies. Recent growth of telecommunications service providers allows health systems and practitioners to purchase only the telemedicine capacity they need. Telemedicine can finance its own investment costs by reducing the cost of care, as telemedicine helps break healthcare's expensive dependency on paper records. Virtual private networks can provide a cost-effective alternative for hospitals linking physicians in a marketwide intranet or a national health system organizing its far-flung hospitals into a privately operated network (Guy 1999). VPNS incur the costs of establishing a complete telecommunications network, from servers and software to security, and assume the responsibility for upgrading the network as new technology becomes available. Few healthcare providers have the scale, technical skills, and capital to match VPNS in a return-on-investment comparison.

10. Security

Consumers are understandably concerned about the privacy of their medical information as hospitals and medical offices convert paper records to electronic formats. Biosensors and software can be used to authenticate the identity of persons seeking access to medical information and to verify their authorization to see it. Electronic medical records systems can document all interactions, including any changes made to the records. Finally, encryption software can render medical information unreadable while it is communicated across the Internet. HIPAA, also known as the Kennedy-Kassebaum Act, was Washington's response to political pressures to protect electronic medical records of patient-identifiable information. HIPAA implementation is now proceeding, five years after enactment. Congress also approved legislation establishing standards for electronic signatures in 2000.

LOOKING FORWARD: THE FUTURE OF TELEMEDICINE

Telemedicine is an emerging technology and innovative health delivery model, but it is still very much a work in progress. Definitive statements about telemedicine in some future year, say 2005 or 2010, would contradict the lessons of its development over the past five to ten years. The technology supporting telemedicine has changed faster than expected, creating unforeseen possibilities along the way. Creative entrepreneurs, many of them physicians, have harnessed this potential by bringing to market new ways of providing healthcare. Visionary executives have crafted unexpected strategic partnerships, finding synergy among companies in different lines of business. Growth in consumer use of the Internet, including e-health services, has been phenomenal and unprecedented. Seldom has a new technology been adopted in the health field so quickly by so many.

Perhaps the most important conclusion is that the convergence of computers and telecommunications offers much more than a new medium in which to deliver traditional healthcare. Telemedicine is creating a whole new concept of healthcare delivery. Progress in the evolution of telemedicine is gaining momentum, and American healthcare is uniquely positioned to exploit its potential. The United States has a unique combination of Internet capacity, telecommunications companies, and innovative provider organizations; on a global basis, low-cost, Internet-enabled telemedicine could revolutionize healthcare. The world is watching to see how the delivery of health and medical care can be improved: telemedicine may offer a world-class solution.

STRATEGIC IMPLICATIONS

Rapid technological progress explains why telemedicine's realm of possibility is expanding at such an amazing rate. Following are some guidelines for dealing with the evolving technologies of telemedicine (Bauer and Ringel 1999, pp. 145–54).

Stay Informed and Open-Minded. With the rapid pace of technological in-novation, what was "true" about telemedicine last year is likely to be different now and irrelevant next year.

Specify the Need, Select the Technology. Early adopters of telemedicine often installed hardware, usually an interactive video system, and then tried to figure out what to do with it. Define the problem, then evaluate the tech-nologies of telemedicine to identify an optimal response.

Consider Outsourcing. In the make-versus-buy equation, outsourcing the technology and telecommunications function may be the most cost-effec-tive solution.

Acquire User-Friendly Systems. Ease of use should be one of the most im-portant design criteria in building telemedicine capability. Consultants sug-gest site visits to evaluate equipment and interview users.

Use an Open Architecture. When building a telemedicine network, make sure that all devices are capable of communicating in a common format, so equipment can be mixed and matched as needed and expanded as tech-nology evolves.

Involve the Customer. Telemedicine's ultimate success will depend on the extent that both providers and patients are comfortable with the technol-ogy and that systems are designed that meet the needs of all parties.

REFERENCES

Bauer, J. C., and R. C. Coile, Jr. 2000. "Should Physicians Be Paid for Online Care? E-Frontier Challenges Traditional Reimbursement." *Medical Crossfire* 2 (10): 1–3.

Bauer, J. C., and M. A. Ringel. 1999. *Telemedicine and the Reinvention of Healthcare: The Seventh Revolution in Medicine.* New York: McGraw-Hill.

Bosak, J., and T. Bray. 1999. "XML and the Second-Generation Web." *Scientific American* May: 89–93.

Galdabini, G. 2000. "First Health to Reimburse Physicians for Patient Consultations over the Internet." *Managed Care Outlook* 13 (19): 1–2.

Guy, S. 1999. "Virtual Private Networks." *American Medical News,* March 1, p. 26.

Kvedar, J. C., E. Menn, and K. R. Loughlin. 1998. "Telemedicine: Present Applications and Future Prospects." *Urologic Clinics of North America* 25 (1): 137–49.

Murphy, R. L., T. B. Fitzpatrick, H. A. Hayes, et al. 1972. "Accuracy of Dermatologic Diagnosis by Television." *Archives of Dermatology* 105 (6): 833–5.

Preston, J. 1999. *The Telemedicine Handbook: Improving Health Care With Interactive Video.* Austin, TX: Telemedical Interactive Consultative Services.

Tieman, J. 2001. "Dialing Up High-Tech Medicine." *Modern Healthcare* 31 (1): 36.

Wheat, H. 2001. "Paying for E-Visits May Become a Trend Among Employers and Health Plans." *Managed Care Outlook* 14 (13): 1, 6.

CHAPTER TEN

Medical Errors and the Science of Care Management

KEY CONCEPTS: *Medical errors • Clinical practice variation • No-fault system • Medications management • Clinical collaboratives • Virtual data warehouse*

INTRODUCTION: The 1999 Institute of Medicine report on medical errors sent a shock wave across the health industry. The report projected that 44,000 to 98,000 patients died needlessly each year in American hospitals due to errors in the process of their treatment. Media attention has continued, and the Institute of Medicine recently called for a national fund of $1 billion to support quality improvement initiatives. The Institute for Healthcare Improvement in Boston, has fostered the development of dozens of "clinical collaboratives" in health systems and regions across the nation. Quality improvement is a business strategy. Case studies in errors reduction and medications management suggest substantial savings of millions can be achieved in typical hospitals. The attention to medical errors is likely to lead to government regulations and mandatory reporting.

"EVEN AS THE debate goes on [in Congress], providers are moving forward quietly to try to improve their medical errors rate, and physicians and physician executives are in the forefront of attempts to change the process of care delivery—and with it, the underlying culture of know-nothingism that has long pervaded American medicine."

—*Mark Haglund (2000, pp. 1, 6)*

Hospitals and doctors were shocked when the Institute of Medicine (IOM) released its report on medical errors in November 1999; it estimated that between 44,000 and 98,000 patients die each year due to errors in hospitals across the United States. Entitled *To Err is Human: Building a Safer Health System,* the report was a devastating critique of American medicine, exposing a pattern of miscommunication and medical blunders even in hospitals at which care was thought to be the "gold standard of the world" (Kohn, Corrigan, and Donaldson 1999). The estimate of 98,000 deaths is higher than that for breast cancer, highway accidents, or AIDS, according to the 223-page report. The federal Department of Health and Human Services has endorsed IOM's goal of reducing errors 50 percent within five years through a combination of research and reporting. Additional funding of $30 to $35 million per year is proposed by IOM for the creation of a federal Center for Patient Safety within the Agency for Healthcare Research and Quality. Grants from this funding would promote development of technology for medical errors reporting. Mandatory reporting for Medicare hospitals is very likely.

Award-winning journalist Michael Millenson also sent a powerful message in his widely read book, *Demanding Medical Excellence,* which warned that the American healthcare experience is far from producing "zero defects." Millenson asks, "Why don't patients typically get the best possible care, and how should the practice of medicine change so that they do?" (Millenson 1997, p. 15). Improving the quality of American medical care is a trend that reflects the growing influence of consumerism. A recent study by Arthur Anderson and the Health Forum, the San Francisco–based division of the American Hospital Association, focused on consumer expectations of the highest quality as one of the key drivers of twenty-first-century healthcare (Geniat and Johnson 2000). Quality, as defined by consumers, includes not only the absence of medical errors, but also addresses the patients' interactions with doctors, support staff, technology, and how the system deals with people. But will the health system respond? The Anderson study found that healthcare leaders were "conflicted" about the issue of customer versus cost. Healthcare executives understand the consumer agenda but tend to rank reducing costs as a higher priority (73 percent) than partnering with employees economically (34 percent).

Medication errors cost an estimated $2,500 to $3,500 per bed per year, according to studies by Superior Consultant in Southfield, Michigan (Zaffrin 2000), a cost that could add up to $1.6 million yearly for a 450-bed hospital. In one pilot study, a large teaching hospital spent $5 million dealing with adverse drug reactions. Where do drug errors take place? More than half occur in ordering, and more than one-third occur in administration, according to assessments in several research studies.

Despite significant capital investments by hospitals in information technology and electronic medical records, quality management experts cite an "analytic gap" as a major reason that clinical care is not better managed and patterns of medical errors are missed (Brailer et al. 1996). In Philadelphia, CareScience has partnered with the University of Pennsylvania to develop the Clinical and Administrative Decision-Support Utility and Clinical Information System (CaduCIS), a care management software package. In a pilot project with the Graduate Health System, care managers identified an unexpectedly high rate of complications in patients with congestive heart failure (CHF). Automating the data analysis reduced the amount of time by a factor of 10:1, time that doctors would have spent in chart review to identify the causes of the complications. Care managers also identified one widely used test in CHF management that had no apparent clinical benefit, saving $8 per test for 3,000 patients per year. The project provides evidence that clinical performance improvement pays off in lower complication rates and associated costs, less use of expensive tests and therapies, and more efficient staff time in problem analysis and improving clinical pathways.

QUALITY IS A BUSINESS STRATEGY

The payoffs from clinical quality improvement could be millions of dollars of eliminated rework, savings which could put every hospital in the United States in the black. The Institute of Medicine estimates the cost of nonfatal medical errors is $17 to $19 billion each year (Rovner 2000). According to IOM, between 2.9 and 3.7 percent of all hospital admissions suffered an injury as a result of medical mismanagement (Benjamin 2000). "Quality is a business strategy" at the Sacred Heart Medical Center in Spokane, Washington (Davis 2000). The hospital has set a three-year, $10 million target for cost reduction by lowering the incidence of medical errors, reported Sacred Heart's Skip Davis at a recent CEO Summit sponsored by Superior Consultant. Working with Bridge Medical, a San Diego–based firm that provides error-reporting software, the hospital believes that 10 to 15 percent of its operating costs involve duplicative rework and complications caused by adverse events, which amounts to as much as $40 to $50 million at Sacred Heart. Bridge Medical estimates a savings of more than $1.6 million at the hospital annually by addressing the problem of medication errors. At a cost of $95 per preventable error and an error rate of one percent, Sacred Heart can significantly lower its costs per discharge with a research and development and information systems investment of less than $500,000. CEO Davis also reports nursing productivity gains of 20 minutes per RN per shift. More good news: the hospital's malpractice insurance costs have been reduced by the carrier by 10 percent.

Providers can learn from other industries about competing on quality. In Chicago, Northwestern Memorial's CEO Gary Mecklenburg argues that hospitals and health systems must overcome their isolation from other industries and learn from the best of the best in the private sector: "Today, healthcare organizations are subject to the same economic forces, the same business principles, and the same standards that exist for the rest of the economy" (Lanser 2000). Mecklenburg invested $580 million in a state-of-the-art, 200 million square foot replacement facility that opened last year. Northwestern's high-visibility commitment to quality is backed up by the hospital's patient-first philosophy. Mecklenburg is delighted when patients say, "this [new facility] doesn't look like a hospital." Northwestern was specifically inspired by the Ritz-Carlton and Disney in developing consumer-centered facilities and systems.

Promising results are being seen from the efforts by a number of provider organizations to systematically reduce medication errors, perhaps the most frequent source of medical mistakes. The Veterans Administration (VA) has installed electronic monitoring systems for medication administration in nearly one in four VA facilities. At the VA pilot site in Topeka, Kansas, the Colmery-O'Neil VA Medical Center experienced a 64 percent reduction in medical errors in comparison with its baseline error rates from 1993, the last year the VA relied on a fully paper-based medication administration system (IHC 2000). In fact, these dramatic results may be understated. VA officials believe that error rates in the past were probably underreported because they relied on people reporting their own mistakes.

IS THE NATION'S HEALTH THREATENED BY MEDICAL ERRORS?

If the IOM study is accurate, the unintended errors of modern hospital care are the equivalent of the crash of a 747 aircraft every day. In the intervening months, the venerable Institute of Medicine has found itself in the middle of a raging debate over the adequacy of the data and the validity of the scientific analyses behind the error study. For example, in the *Journal of the American Medical Association,* critics of the study shot back with an article entitled, "Deaths Due to Medical Errors Are Exaggerated in Institute of Medicine Report" (McDonald, Weiner, and Hui 2000). They argue that today's hospitalized patients have "high disease burdens and high death risks," suggesting that most in-hospital deaths will occur regardless of how many "accidents" are avoided. In a similar article in the *New England Journal of Medicine,* a physician from Boston-based Brigham & Women's Hospital cautions that "careful readers must have some reservations" about the IOM report (Brennan 2000).

The Institute of Medicine report has outraged consumer organizations and health insurers, who are calling for new federal legislation to require mandatory reporting of medical mishaps. Congressional proposals have centered on a no-fault system like that used by pilots to report safety lapses and in-air near misses. The American Hospital Association and American Medical Association have been highly vocal in their rejection of mandatory reporting and increased federal oversight. They fear that making error data public will expose hospitals and doctors to a flurry of lawsuits.

A federal bureaucracy is already being established that could provide oversight for a national program in medical errors. AHRQ has the Congressional mandate to provide leadership in error reporting and process improvement. The Agency spent much of the 1990s developing medical practice guidelines, but heavy opposition from the American Medical Association and other medical groups curbed the federal initiatives for defining national standards of practice. Dr. John Eisenberg, the Agency's director, chairs the federal Quality Interagency Coordination Task Force, created by the Clinton administration in 1998.

MEDICATION MANAGEMENT

The implementation of a medication management solution with built-in quality checks will help organizations reduce their incidence of medical mistakes—specifically, medication errors—while reducing associated costs with managing medication inventory. Preventable adverse drug events occur at four stages (Bates et al. 1995):

1. Ordering by physician—56 percent of medication errors: wrong dose, wrong choice of drug, patient has a known allergy to the drug.
2. Administration of medication orders by nursing staff—34 pecent of medication errors: wrong drug, wrong dose of drug administered, wrong time, wrong technique used to administer drug.
3. Transcription of medication order by secretarial staff—6 percent of medication errors: wrong frequency of drug administration, missed dose because medication is not transcribed.
4. Dispensation of medications ordered by the pharmacy department—4 percent of medication errors: wrong time (drug not

sent in time to be given to patient at time ordered), wrong drug, wrong dose.

The medication management process in hospitals has not evolved to the same degree technologically as other clinical processes. Today's processes rely heavily on oral or written communication among various clinicians and administrative personnel across various functions within the hospital. The medication management process affects registrars, physicians, nurses, pharmacists, finance, quality or risk management staff, materials management personnel, and the patient, with many activities taking place far from the bedside. A process of this complexity poses significant opportunities for error. The medication management process begins at the time the patient is admitted or enters the enterprise; includes processes associated with medication ordering, transcription, and dispensing; and continues with administering and documenting medications given to patients, as well as posting charges, updating inventory, and replenishing stock. Quality and risk management processes are affected retrospectively when errors occur. In a pilot project in a North Carolina medical center, point-of-care systems for positive bar code identification resulted in significant improvements in medications processes, including a 52 percent reduction in doses omitted, a 43 percent decrease in medications delivered at the wrong time, and a 33 percent drop in the wrong drugs being administered (Zaffrin 2000).

Medication management solutions in their ultimate implementation address all the components of the process, including

- ordering;
- clinical checking;
- drug distribution;
- automated drug dispensing device (e.g., PYXIS) interfaces;
- point-of-care positive patient-drug identification via bar code;
- documentation of medication administration;
- charge capture based on administration;

- supply-chain management; and
- error and outcomes analysis.

Studies have shown that about 35 percent of all medication errors occur at the point of administration. This is a step in the process that until recently was not easy to automate, track, or quality ensure. Advancements in radio-frequency networks and mobile computing capabilities are making point-of-care devices and bar code technology more acceptable to the healthcare industry. This technology now makes verification of the right drug for the right patient possible prior to administration, at the point of care. The combination of high-tech devices, the ability to eliminate serious medication errors, and quality assurance have become the highlight features of medication management offerings. Although technology alone is not a medication management solution, it has become the focus of many vendors who seek to integrate technology into their existing medication management components.

QUESTIONS ABOUT PRACTICE VARIATIONS

Variation in clinical practice is a national challenge for healthcare providers and purchasers. The *Dartmouth Atlas of Health Care,* developed by the Center for Evaluative Clinical Sciences of the Dartmouth Medical School, has made a science of the "geography of healthcare" in the United States (Dartmouth 2000). In collaboration with the American Hospital Association, researchers at Dartmouth are committed to the establishment of a new model of clinical decision making that applies benchmarks of performance. The *Atlas* was written by a remarkable father-son team, Dr. John Wennberg, director of Dartmouth Medical School's Center for Evaluative Health Sciences, and son David Wennberg, M.D., director of the Center for Outcomes Research and Evaluation at the Maine Medical Center.

For a variety of major conditions, the Dartmouth *Atlas* is vivid proof that dozens of local medical markets experience 30 percent higher use rates than the national average, whereas many other regions are lower than national benchmarks. The *Atlas* relies on a 20 percent sample of

Table 10.1: Report Card on Cost of Six Months at End of Life (Medicare Data)

Metropolitan Area	Cost of Care in Last Six Months of Life
Manhattan, NY	$16,571
Miami, FL	$14,212
Chicago, IL	$12,543
Philadelphia, PA	$12,093
Los Angeles, CA	$11,800
Milwaukee, WI	$ 8,007
Seattle, WA	$ 7,255
Minneapolis, MN	$ 7,246
Portland, OR	$ 6,793

Source: Dartmouth (2000, p. 95).

Medicare patients, based on a national small-area analysis of 313 hospital referral regions. Costs of care in the last six months of life were found to vary tremendously (see Table 10.1). For example, use of intensive care in the last six months varies for no apparent medical or demographic reason. In Newark, New Jersey, 41.5 percent of dying patients were cared for in an ICU, as were 47.5 percent of patients in Miami, Florida, but only 26.8 percent in Milwaukee, Wisconsin, and 25.0 percent in Seattle, Washington, of terminal patients were given the costly treatment of intensive care.

Researchers at Dartmouth found in many local markets that variations are more common than similarities in clinical practice. In Louisiana, the referral rate for radical prostatectomies in Baton Rouge is 4.9 procedures per 1,000 population, the highest in the nation; in nearby Lafayette, the rate is 0.9 per 1,000, the lowest. In terms of medical procedures, data from the Dartmouth *Atlas* suggest that "geography is destiny," according to Dr. Jack Lord, former chief operating officer for the American Hospital Association, which publishes the *Atlas* (Moore 1998, p. 104). The *Atlas* also demonstrates that the more hospital beds in the local market, the higher the use rates and health costs are likely to be. Louisiana, whose hospital bed-to-patient ratio is in the highest quintile, is also one of the highest-cost states, where an above-average number of Medicare patients die in hospitals. These large swings in use rates and health costs found in the *Atlas* suggest wasted resources and opportunities for clinical cost management for every hospital and health system in the United States.

Employers are taking on the issue of clinical variation and quality improvement as a major factor in driving up health benefits costs. In three metropolitan areas, coalitions of major employers are underwriting a regional assessment of clinical variation in patterns—and costs—of care (White 1999). Chicago's Jim Mortimer, president of the Midwest Business Group on Health, notes that the Dartmouth *Atlas* data "can raise red flags for employers" by displaying how their markets differ significantly from other similar regions. Major differences provide clues to employer-backed quality improvement initiatives. The Midwest Business Group, in partnership with the American Hospital Association's Health Research and Educational Trust and the Robert Wood Johnson Foundation is conducting three demonstration projects in Muncie, Indiana; Milwaukee; and Witchita, Kansas, which bring together employers with local hospitals and doctors to determine the causes for clinical and cost variation in their communities. In Muncie, for example, attention focused on the high rate for angioplasty, in comparison with a similar region, South Bend, Indiana. After seeing the data, Muncie physicians are doing a better job of advising their patients on alternatives to angioplasty.

PROVIDERS RESPOND WITH QUALITY INITIATIVES

Providers are responding to the IOM report with publicity and process improvement procedures. The Boston-based Institute for Healthcare Improvement produced a report in February 2000 called, "Reducing Medical Errors and Improving Patient Safety: Success Stories from the Front Lines of Medicine" (Haglund 2000). Led by Dr. Donald Berwick, the Institute has pioneered quality improvement efforts for 20 years. At the St. Louis, Missouri–based SSM Health Care system, Dr. Andrew

Kosseff, an internist, has taken the lead in a year-long "clinical collaboratives" project, inspired by the Institute for Healthcare Improvement. SSM's initiative covers 21 hospitals in four states. Three projects are currently under way, including prescribing practices, secondary prevention of ischemic heart disease, and using patient information to improve healthcare delivery.

In Salt Lake City, Utah, the InterMountain Health System has relentlessly pursued a program of clinical process improvement for more than a decade. Dr. Brent James, vice president for medical research, reports a 75 percent improvement in the drug error rate and in reducing quality problems at the system's flagship LDS Hospital (Haglund 2000). Problems such as patient falls, nosocomial infections, decubitus ulcers, blood transfusion errors, and pulmonary embolisms arising from deep vein thrombosis have been targets for clinical process management. But further improvements in quality are possible. When InterMountain applied intensive computer analysis to drug errors at LDS, it found 80 times more adverse drug events, but few hospitals have the databases and tools to assess such data.

Hospitals are adding quality indicators to their dashboard reports of key benchmarks of organizational performance. At a recent conference for strategic planners and marketing executives sponsored by Rand Healthcare Roundtables of Thousand Oaks, California, several provider initiatives in constructing management dashboards were profiled by Howard Gershon of Arista Associates, a healthcare consulting firm based in Chicago and Washington, DC. At the St. Lukes Regional Medical Center in Boise, Idaho, the board of directors took the lead in asking management to give them a snapshot of the business in a continuing report series (O'Keeffe 2000). The 14-factor report includes such quality indicators as ER treatment times, patient satisfaction, perioperative deaths, and unscheduled readmissions. The results are presented in full-color reports in which green indicators are above-goal levels and red data indicate below-goal performance. Wausau-based Community Health Care, a regional health system in central Wisconsin, has used dashboard indicators for five years (Day 2000). Wausau's report was inspired by the Juran Institute and updates critical performance measures monthly. Thirteen indicators provide the board and management with continuous updates on growth, performance, and service and quality, including patient occurrences per 1,000 days, number of customer complaints, patient satisfaction, and readmissions with three days per 1,000 discharges.

The Medical Group Management Association (MGMA) is one of the leaders in physician efforts to address the problem of errors in medical practice. Dr. William Jessee, MGMA president and CEO, calls the IOM report "an issue that has long deserved attention" (Haglund 2000, p. 9). MGMA has a four-pronged effort under way to promote patient safety with its 20,000-member group practices.

The improvement from electronic monitoring of medication errors is raising issues for VA managers (IHC 2000), who now find themselves grappling with whether to revise their traditional policy of disciplining nurses who make several errors. At the national level, VA headquarters discourages discipline on the basis of error rates, but local VA facilities have discretion.

SEVEN STEPS TOWARD QUALITY IMPROVEMENT

Consumer advocates and the media are asking the question, "Why is there so much variation in medicine when we have so much evidence as to what works?" (Weber 2000a, p. 14). There is no short answer to that question. Given the publicity of the Institute of Medicine findings, many hospitals and physician groups will focus on the immediate issue of medical errors. Placing a high management priority on clinical improvement is much more than reducing medical errors. A synergy exists among the elements of quality improvement, disease management, clinical efficiency, and patient satisfaction. At the Lovelace Health System in Albuquerque, New Mexico, a disease management program for clinical depression saved $1 million (Reeder 2000). A similar program is under way in San Diego at the Sharp Health System, with a goal to improve the underdiagnosis of depression in patients who are presenting themselves to the health system for a variety of other ailments, such as chest and back pain.

The following are seven successful strategies for reducing medical errors and improving clinical performance.

1. Science of Error Reduction

A new "science of errors" is needed to track deviations from standards and benchmarks and probe lapses of care, such as nosocomial infections, patient falls, and medication errors (Weber 2000a). Quality experts cite the airlines as a responsive industry, which has moved aggressively to prevent pilot and air traffic control errors that could lead to fatal crashes. Three ingredients are essential to making systematic progress in the science of errors: (1) a no-fault error-reporting system that records a high percentage of all errors; (2) extensive computerized databases of clinical performance with IT-facilitated data analysis; and (3) a management process for disseminating information and improving clinical performance.

Hospitals should develop a voluntary reporting system of medical errors in the short term. Hospital and health system administrators are advised to find out how large a problem the organization may have now and develop an error reduction plan. They should also prepare for the likelihood of mandatory reporting, which could be imposed by government within the next two to three years. Furthermore, states may not wait for Washington, DC, to enact their own error oversight legislation. The State of Massachusetts has created a coalition to examine ways to prevent medical errors, and Maryland's Health Care Commission has also begun to investigate hospital quality.

In Michigan, the Borgess Medical Center of Kalamazoo was dismayed to discover a much higher than expected mortality rate for nonsurgical heart cases (CareScience 2000). According to data published annually by the Michigan Hospital Association, the hospital's mortality data were above expected benchmark levels. Cardiology is a major service line for Borgess, which is nationally recognized as one of the top 100 hospitals for interventional cardiology, but the nonsurgical mortality experience for a group of 15 diagnosis-related groups (DRGS) and 1,500 patients was unexpectedly high. In response, the hospital brought in Caducis.com and its Institute for Management Development, a division of CareScience, a Philadelphia-based quality management consulting firm that developed the Caduscis risk assessment methodology. Three DRGs for management of acute miocardial infarction (AMI) were found to account for the greatest deviation from risk-adjusted predicted mortality. The researchers recommended a number of actions, including targeting noncardiologists for continuing medical education in the latest treatment protocols, such as use of beta-blockers. In the three-month period following the implementation of improvement strategies for AMI patients, the mortality rate decreased from 19 percent to 8 percent.

2. Electronic Medical Records

The electronic medical record is much more than an automated paper record. It is a database and decision-support system. In California's trend-setting San Diego market, the Sharp Healthcare System believes that investing in electronic medical records is a fundamental key to gaining efficiency and restoring financial profitability. Taking the waste out of clinical processes can generate significant return on investment for Sharp's four general acute hospitals, three specialty facilities, and three large affiliated medical groups (Reeder 2000). John Byrnes, M.D., Sharp's senior vice president for clinical effectiveness, was formerly responsible for the extensive clinical engineering and benchmarking program at Albuquerque's Lovelace Clinic. He is now overseeing the installation of an electronic medical records system at Sharp. In the intensively competitive San Diego market, with one of the highest managed care penetration rates in the nation, Byrnes believes it is "absolutely imperative that in addition to delivering quality care, we be able to prove that we can deliver quality care" (Reeder 2000, p. 7).

Collecting data about the frequency, nature, and severity of errors is essential in order to create a baseline, record deviations from standards and procedures, and analyze performance over time. A number of healthcare organizations are moving their electronic medical records and other health-related information into large, multiaccess data warehouses. The concept of a shared data warehouse is highly useful for integrated health systems that want to link their physicians to ambulatory, in-patient, and long-term-care units with a common data repository and retrieval system.

A new concept now in pilot testing works like a "virtual data warehouse." In Santa Barbara, a consortium of Medicaid providers is working with CareScience of Philadelphia to create the Care Data Exchange program (Morrisey 2000). The three-year demonstration project is funded in part by a $10 million grant from the California HealthCare Foundation, with all participants investing another $20 million to develop the protocols and infrastructure. The concept is simple: All participants hold their own data but set up common interchange standards and protocols. The Care Data Exchange project links a countywide network of hospitals and physicians with the Santa Barbara Health Department, Blue Cross, and other Medicaid-participating managed care organizations. Any participant can request and receive information from any other participant. Protocols protect patient privacy and security. All data exchanges are confidential, and some data cannot be shared without the patient's permission. No data are transferred except by specific and authorized request, and no centralized warehouse of information exists to be maintained or managed. Although the project is only in the early stages of implementation, it is already attracting attention from a number of other potential users and applications.

3. Design Around Patients

Design clinical improvement programs around patients, not providers. The baseline for successful disease management programs is patient-centered care, believes Dr. John Byrnes, who was responsible for developing the award-winning disease management programs at the Lovelace Health System (Reeder 2000). According to the Lovelace experience, when clinical performance improvement programs are designed to respond to the needs and wants of patients, patient satisfaction ratings "go through the roof." Physicians and nursing staff respond to the positive aspirations of patient-centered clinical processes, and the perception of quality ripples across the organization and into the community.

Table 10.2: VA Medication Error Reduction

Error Reduction Strategy	Percent Improvement
Wrong time incidents	91.6
Wrong patient incidents	91.3
Wrong medication incidents	73.8
Omitted doses	69.6
Wrong dose incidents	56.6

Source: IHC (2000).

4. Reducing Medication Errors

The biggest target for immediate quality improvement may be reducing medication errors. In pilot projects for error reduction, San Diego–based Bridge Medical, a quality improvement management firm, has found that hospitals may have at least a one percent medication error rate (Davis 2000). Some facilities may err in as many as 3 to 4 percent of all medication transactions, including wrong drug, wrong dose, wrong time, patient allergy, omitted medication, and drug incompatibility with other medications. Drug waste is another form of medication error, when costly drugs are allowed to expire and are ultimately disposed of by nursing staff or taken off shelves by hospital pharmacists (Lang 2000a).

To respond to these issues, the Department of Veterans Affairs is rolling out a VA-developed wireless point-of-care medication administration system. The new system has already been installed in 37 VA facilities, with a 64.5 percent reduction in medical errors in the Colmery-O'Neil VA Medical Center in Topeka, Kansas (IHC 2000). Errors were reduced in a variety of ways (see Table 10.2) when the VA shifted from a paper-based system to electronic monitoring of medications. VA nurses use computers mounted on medication carts in a number of sites; other facilities use a separate cart. The prototype was built by Colmery-O'Neil with assistance from EDS in developing the final code.

5. Research Organization

Quality experts recommend the creation of a dedicated research organization, which can integrate data and manage the process of disseminating information. Douglas Thompson suggests development of an RIID (report, investigate, innovate, and disseminate) unit (Thompson 2000). This is a cross-functional team similar to quality improvement (QI) programs in place in many hospitals and health systems, which applies systematic and multidisciplinary analysis to error reduction, relying on information systems to a much greater extent than traditional QI efforts.

Much more could be done to systematically upgrade clinical quality and reduce clinical variation with greater research and development (R&D) commitment and resources. For instance, quality experts believe that clinical improvement research is underfunded among hospitals and health systems (Weber 2000a). At California-based Kaiser Permanente, Joe Selby, director of research, receives only $3 million of his $21 million R&D budget from inside the Kaiser system. The Kaiser R&D program is one of the most extensive in the industry; barely two dozen of the nation's 600 HMOs have an organized health services research program. At the University of California San Francisco Medical Center, clinicians Robert Wachter, M.D., and colleague Lee Goldman, M.D., were turned down by two foundations and the federal government when they sought research funding to compare the costs and outcomes of in-patient care directed by primary care physicians versus hospitalists. The doctors eventually paid for the evaluation out of their departmental budget and validated the hospitalist concept in an influential article in the *New England Journal of Medicine* (Wachter and Goldman 2000).

Multiorganizational collaboratives are a low-cost, highly practical strategy for harnessing provider organizations in the real work of clinical process improvement. The collaborative approach is encouraged by the Boston-based Institute for Healthcare Improvement, led by Donald Berwick, M.D., a widely respected leader of clinical quality improvement efforts for more than two decades (Lang 2000b). The collaborative approach is a learning laboratory in which participants meet to benchmark performance and share results about what works, in projects lasting 6 to 18 months. Peer-to-peer competition among the participants can be a powerful motivator for improvement, say collaborative organizers. In St. Louis, SSM Health Care, a 21-hospital system, has three internal collaboratives in process, with plans for five more within the next 18 months. California-based Catholic Healthcare West has 15 of its 46 hospitals participating in an internal collaborative on care of patients with community-acquired pneumonia.

6. Chronic Illness Focus

There is a good reason to focus care management and error reduction programs on chronically ill patients: The "right care to the right patient at the right time" can be the most cost-effective strategy for reforming healthcare in the United States (Rauber 1999). Those with chronic health conditions are the most frequent customers of the nation's $1.3 trillion health system. The United States spends about $400 billion— one dollar in three—on care of chronically ill patients who are the targets for systematic disease management. For example, diabetics make up 5 percent of the population but consume 14 percent of all health expenditures. Early identification and management of diabetes can prevent kidney damage, avoiding $70,000 per year for renal dialysis or $100,000 for a kidney transplant.

Health plans are taking aim at chronic conditions. At Cigna, pilot programs in asthma, diabetes, and lower back pain have been so successful that they are being expanded nationwide (Rauber 1999). Humana is focusing its care management programs on 40,000 of its 6.2 million enrollees, those at highest risk—and whose care will be most expensive—with conditions such as congestive heart failure, asthma, and cancer as well as those newborns in need of intensive care. In Iowa, Wellmark, which operates the Blue Cross plan, has found that 20 percent of its enrollees account for 87 percent of the health plan's medical costs, and just one percent of Wellmark's patients were responsible for $465 million of the $1.5 billion the plan spent on healthcare benefits in 2000. The health plans' challenge is to encourage their

Table 10.3: National Quality Benchmarks from the Top-Ranked 100 Hospitals

Performance Measure	National Benchmark	Peer Group Average
Mortality index	0.86	1.00
Complications index	0.57	0.66
Severity-adjusted length of stay	4.12	4.44

Source: *Modern Healthcare* (2001).

networks' physicians to eliminate unexplained clinical variation and consistently follow the best accepted medical practices. Many plans are engaged in extensive profiling of physician performance in managing high-cost conditions. The plans insist they are not exercising "economic credentialing," but many insurers and managed care organizations such as Minneapolis-based United are producing care management report cards that advise doctors of their status in comparison with national benchmarks.

7. Link to Financial Performance

It is clear from the annual analysis of the top 100 hospitals in the nation that the payoff from clinical performance improvement is better financial results (Weber 2000b). These hospitals achieve top performance in eight key indicators of clinical quality, operational efficiency, and financial strength; three factors relate directly to quality: (1) risk-adjusted mortality index, (2) risk-adjusted complications index, and (3) severity-adjusted average length of stay (see Table 10.3).

Staying in the top 100 is getting tougher. Peer group institutions are improving their quality, while leading facilities are experiencing a tailing-off in mortality and complication rates. In 1999, length of stay dropped only fractionally, from 4.18 to 4.12 days, which was still better than the peer-group average of 4.44 days.

Clinical efficiency directly contributes to financial success. Top-100 hospitals averaged a total profit margin of 8.71 percent, considerably more profitable than their peers, who made only 1.88 percent total net margin in the HCIA-Sachs assessment.

InterMountain's Dr. Brent James states his organization's case for investing in clinical performance improvement: "Our competitive advantage arises from implementation [of R&D findings]. Because we do the research, we see the results earlier. We figure there is a 2–4 year lag, even if you're being entirely open about it, before the rest of the world gets a look" (Weber 2000a). At Sacramento, California–based Sutter Health System, CEO Van Johnson, a former InterMountain executive, earmarked $650,000 to establish the Sutter Health Institute for Research and Education. Sutter's R&D organization is receiving a commitment of 16 percent of the health system's $4 million bottom line last year, with million dollar funding in future years. Johnson is convinced that research and education around clinical improvement will boost his organization finances, arguing "we could achieve as much total improvement in the health of this nation from executing consistently what we already know about how to deliver state-of-the-art medical care, as we are likely to receive from all the recent advances in human genetic and pharmaceutical research" (Weber 2000a, p. 60).

WHY QUALITY IMPROVEMENT EFFORTS SOMETIMES FAIL

Many hospitals and health systems have initiated quality improvement, but often with mixed results. At the University of Pennsylvania Health System in Philadelphia, chief medical officer David Shulkin, M.D., identifies a number of failings that can reduce the effectiveness of quality initiatives (Shulkin 2000):

- too many meetings;
- overemphasis on process;
- need for incentives;
- organizational and personality barriers;

- too much data;
- relying on outside benchmarks;
- no accountability for results;
- too long a time line;
- too many QI projects; and
- not knowing when to call it quits.

Underinvestment in information technology is another limiting factor. Mark Leavitt, chairman of Medscape, complains that healthcare organizations spend only 3.9 percent of their budgets on information technology, in comparison with banking, which spends more than 10 percent and has automated many routine processes (Tedeschi 2000). Medicare budget cuts and managed care have slashed many hospitals' capital budgets, deferring investment in IS and IT upgrades. In Boston, the University of Massachusetts (UMass) Medical Center has invested more than $40 million in information technology over the past five years but is a long way from putting Palm-type electronic medical records in the hands of its doctors. At UMass, the information system does not have enough capacity for x-rays and digital images to be sent across the hospital's network. Only the intensive care unit and emergency department have that capability. "We lose money on every admission," notes a UMass senior executive. The hospital will focus on technology upgrades this year but cannot afford Windows 2000. This is far from the vision of e-health that drives the hospital's information technology managers, but it is the reality until more capital becomes available.

LOOKING FORWARD: OVERCOMING THE CULTURE OF COLLEGIAL SELF-PROTECTION

The Institute of Medicine study is a caution light for America's surging $1.3 trillion health industry. Critics warn that hospitalization could be "hazardous to your health," noting that in a three-day stay, the odds are one in five that a caregiver will make a mistake that harms a patient (Dutton 2000). Even more alarming is the fact that in the face of

estimates that 44,000 to 98,000 deaths may result from medical errors, only 655 errors have voluntarily been reported to JCAHO since
1995. Insurance executives estimate that less than one percent of all
medical mistakes ever result in a malpractice claim.

Despite the prestige of the Institute of Medicine, many obstacles
lie in the path of clinical outcomes improvement. Lack of data, nationally recognized benchmarks, and analytical software are obvious
problems. But the most difficult hurdle may be cultural—the "don't
ask, don't tell" attitude of many physicians and nurses in the face of
errors by their colleagues. The public's expectation of medicine is simple—zero defects. Doctors or nurses who commit errors face a potential gauntlet of litigation and adverse publicity, which can be career limiting. Today's health system assumes our caregivers are infallible, and
that is the popular expectation. Hospital and medical group managers'
expectations are equally high, meaning no mistakes are allowed. It is
no surprise that hospital workers and doctors tend to hide their errors.
A no-blame environment is needed in which hospitals, physicians, and
employees may report mishaps in an error-reduction process, rather
than a search for the guilty.

Physicians are moving out of a "show-me-the-evidence" phase into
a more constructive "how-can-I-use-the-evidence" phase, according to
organizers of multiorganizational collaboratives of the type encouraged
by the Boston-based Institute for Healthcare Improvement (Lang
2000b). InterMountain's Dr. Brent James believes that "the shift we
have to make is away from this culture of blame. If you pay any attention to the literature at all, you quickly realize that humans are inher-
ently fallible, regardless of training, knowledge and expertise. The only
way to prevent errors is to establish systems .... The climate must be
changed in order to expose and correct problems in a non-blaming environment" (Haglund 2000).

Federal regulations mandating the reporting of medical errors are
very likely in the near future. Public disclosure is certainly a motivator for change. When hospitals and their physicians are compared side-
by-side with their peers and against national benchmarks, the resulting publicity will drive many providers to significantly improve their

care management systems. The private sector and major employers can play an important role, as well. The goal of projects like that in Muncie, Indiana, in reducing clinical variation will have a long-term payoff for employers and employees in terms of better patient outcomes and lower employer health costs.

The United States has the best patient care in the world, but not all patients are getting it. Reducing clinical variation and medical errors would do much to elevate America's standing in world health comparisons and to slow the rise in health expenditures in the coming years.

STRATEGIC IMPLICATIONS

Recognize the Quality Issue. The demand for accountability and quality improvement is sweeping healthcare, and resulting federal and state legislation is likely. Employers have taken the initiative and threaten to channel their employees to those hospitals and doctors who have the highest quality and lowest error rates. Providers should initiate an information and education campaign to inform the board, medical staff, and management team about quality improvement programs.

Monitor Quality as a Key Benchmark. Establish a widely recognized set of clinical performance measures and report on them regularly. The board, medical staff, and management team should be as focused on clinical quality as they are on financial performance.

Engage in and Fund Clinical Collaboratives. Cooperate in clinical collaboratives for quality improvement in joint projects with peers and competitors. Improving quality is one arena in which every provider can find common ground. The Boston-based Institute for Healthcare Improvement is an excellent resource for managing clinical collaboratives. These projects should have the organization's highest priority and are worthwhile targets for funding by the hospital's or system's foundation.

REFERENCES

Bates, D. W., D. J. Cullen, J. Cooper, H. J. Demonaco, T. Gallivan, R. Hallisey, J. Ives, N. Laird and G. Caffel. 1995. "Incidence of Adverse Drug Events and Potential Adverse Drug Events. Implications for Prevention." ADE Prevention Study Group. *Journal of the American Medical Association* 274: 29–34.

Benjamin, G. C. 2000. "Addressing Medical Errors: The Key to a Safer Health Care System." *Physician Executive* 26 (2): 66–67.

Brailer, D. J., S. Goldfarb, M. Horgan, F. Katz, R. A. Paulus, and K. Zakrewski. 1996. "Improving Performance with Clinical Decision Support." *Journal on Quality Improvement* 22 (7): 443–56.

Brennan, T. A. 2000. "The Institute of Medicine Report on Medical Errors— Could It Do Harm?" *New England Journal of Medicine* 342 (15): 1123–25.

CareScience. 2000. "Public Report Spurs Mortality Reduction at Borgess Medical Center," pp. 1–4. Philadelphia, PA: CareScience.

Dartmouth Medical School. 2000. *The Dartmouth Atlas of Health Care in the United States,* pp. 1–306. Chicago: American Hospital Association.

Davis, S. 2000. "Quality: Our Business Strategy Using New Technology." Presentation, CEO Summit, Superior Consultant, Chicago, October 5, pp. 1–9.

Day, K. L. 2000. "Critical Performance Measures for Wausau Hospital." Presentation, Rand Healthcare Roundtable, Chicago, October 27, pp. 1–21.

Dutton, G. 2000. "Do American Hospitals Get Away with Murder?" *Business & Health* 18 (4): 38–47.

Geniat, E. J., and K. E. Johnson. 2000. *Leadership for a Healthy 21st Century,* pp. 1–28. Chicago: American Hospital Association.

Haglund, M. 2000. "Medical Errors: While the Policy Debate Rages, Clinician Leaders Quietly Push the Healthcare System Toward Quality Improvement." *Physician Performance & Payment Report* 2 (7): 1, 6–10.

Inside Healthcare Computing (IHC). 2000. "VA: Meds System Cut Errors 64% vs. Paper." *Inside Healthcare Computing* 10 (17): 1–2.

Kohn, L., J. Corrigan, and M. Donaldson. 1999. *To Err Is Human: Building A Safer Health System.* Institute of Medicine Report. Washington, DC: National Academy Press.

Lang, M. 2000a. "Hospitals Target High-Cost, High-Volume Medications to Achieve Cost Efficiencies." COR *Clinical Excellence* 1 (2): 1–3.

————. 2000b. "Collaboratives Are the Hot Ticket to Success with Performance Improvement Initiatives." *Healthcare Leadership Review* 19 (9): 1.

Lanser, E. G. 2000. "Lessons from the Business Side of Healthcare." *Healthcare Executive* September/October: 14–19.

McDonald, C. J., M. Weiner, and S. L. Hui. 2000. "Deaths Due to Medical Errors Are Exaggerated in Institute of Medicine Report." *Journal of the American Medical Association* 284 (1): 93–94.

Millenson, M. L. 1997. *Demanding Medical Excellence: Doctors and Accountability in the Information Age.* Chicago: University of Chicago Press.

Modern Healthcare. 2001. "Top 100 Hospitals National Benchmarks." *Modern Healthcare* February 26 (Special Suppl.): 1–40.

Moore, J. D., Jr. 1998. "No Answer Book: Atlas Raises Questions About Practice Variations." *Modern Healthcare* 28 (26): 104.

Morrisey, J. 2000. "Calif. Community Buys into Internet." *Modern Healthcare* 30 (5, Eye on Info. Suppl.): 20.

O'Keeffe, M. 2000. "Measuring for Success." Presentation, Rand Healthcare Roundtable, Chicago, October 27, pp. 1–7.

Rauber, C. 1999. "Disease Management Can Be Good for What Ails Patients and Insurers." *Modern Healthcare* March 29: 48.

Reeder, L. 2000. "Implementing Performance Improvement in Health Systems." *Healthcare Leadership & Management Report* 8 (7): 1–7.

Rovner, J. 2000. "Washington Wakes Up to Medical Mistakes." *Business & Health* 18 (1): 19.

Shulkin, D. J. 2000. "Commentary: Why Quality Improvement Efforts in Healthcare Fail and What Can Be Done About It." *American Journal of Medical Quality* 15 (2): 49–53.

Tedeschi, B. 2000. "No Fun for Sisyphus: The Woes of WebMD and Medscape." *New York Times,* October 25, p. E12.

Thompson, D. 2000. "An Information Systems Strategy for Preventing Medical Errors." *IT Health Strategies* 2 (5): 4.

Wachter, R., and L. Goldman. 2000. "Hospitalists Redefine the Future of Medicine." *Health Trends* September.

Weber, D. O. 2000a. "Confronting the R&D Imperative." *Health Forum Journal* 43 (4): 13–15, 60.

———. 2000b. "The View from the Top: What It Takes to Make HCIA's 100 Top Ranking Hospitals." *Strategies for Healthcare Excellence* 13 (7): 1–12.

White, R. 1999. "Projects Aim to Improve Care: Health Data Compared." *Business Insurance*, January 11, p. 2.

Zaffrin, S. 2000. "Medication Management: Providing End-to-End Solutions for Healthcare Issues." Powerpoint presentation, Superior Consultant, Southfield, MI, October.

CHAPTER ELEVEN

HIPAA, Electronic Privacy, and Internet Transactions

KEY CONCEPTS: *HIPAA* • *Electronic privacy* • *EDI standards* • *Electronic fraud detection systems* • *PKI* • *WEDI*

INTRODUCTION: Under provisions of HIPAA, the Health Insurance Portability and Accountability Act of 1996, federal rules were released in 2001 which require compliance within two years. The original goal of the Kennedy-Kassebaum legislation was to facilitate electronic commerce and reduce the cost of processing medical claims. The federal legislation has also become a major vehicle for protecting patient privacy and ensuring the security of electronic medical records. HIPAA will address the lack of electronic standards for data interchange in healthcare which has hampered the widespread deployment of e-commerce. For consumers, the new federal regulations will compel hospitals, physician offices, health plans, pharmacies, third-party intermediaries, claims clearinghouses, and any other entities that electronically store or transmit health-related information to protect patient privacy, as well as to utilize common electronic standards and interchange protocols. Achieving HIPAA compliance will yield substantial e-commerce as well as cost-reduction benefits for those entities that take a strategic stance toward implementation. The federal government estimates the savings from HIPAA implementation at $29.9 billion over ten years, with an implementation price tag of $17.6 billion, but providers and health plans are highly skeptical of these figures.

"WE HAVE TO surrender some privacy to capture the benefits of information technology. And we have to sacrifice some of the efficiency that electronic sharing of information might produce in order to protect our privacy."

—Wall Street Journal (2001, p. A1)

The World Wide Web is the last frontier of communication and commerce on a global basis; "www" could also stand for "wild, wild West." More than 20 years after being launched as the ARPANET to connect scientists and the military, the Internet is still subject to few rules and regulations. As the influence of the Internet rapidly widens into every sector of commerce and society, consumer advocates and government regulators are making a case that the Internet needs to move beyond its communal roots of self-governance. Key issues that stakeholders in electronic healthcare want addressed include privacy, reliability of consumer and professional health information, and protection against fraud and abuse on the Internet (Fried 2001). New government regulations are gradually intruding into cyberspace, although much of the Internet's traffic is essentially unmonitored and ungoverned.

Health and medicine may be one of the first sectors of the Internet to be extensively regulated. Government protection issues cover a number of areas of concern, such as:

- confidentiality of electronic medical records;
- privacy of health insurance claims transactions;
- electronic transfer of medical and claims data;
- patients' consent to access of their medical records;
- ownership of hospital and physician office records;
- employer inquiries regarding workers' or applicants' health histories; and
- standardization of electronic transactions in medicine.

Electronic medical records may not be very secure. Public concerns about the security of patient records were heightened in December 2000, when a sophisticated Internet hacker took command of large portions of the University of Washington Medical Center's internal information network and downloaded more than 4,000 patient records. The hacker, a Dutch self-employed security consultant, indicated that he executed the break-in to demonstrate the inadequacy of protections for medical records. For more than a month, the hacker was able to intrude into the system, accessing files regarding cardiac and rehabilitation patients, as well as five months of admission and discharge records. The intrusion alarmed University officials when the hacker reported that "all the machines were exposed without any firewalls at all" (Poulsen 2000).

Privacy on the Internet has become a hot-button issue for lawmakers and consumers (Simpson 2001). Hoping to head off dozens of privacy bills in Congress, a new formation of information industry companies, the Online Privacy Alliance—which includes Microsoft, AOL Time Warner, IBM, and AT&T—released four studies showing that Internet privacy regulations would cost billions annually (wsj.com 2001). With web sites compiling vast databases on their visitors, pressure is mounting for new legislation to limit Internet firms from selling consumers' information without their consent. In a survey of Internet users by the Harris organization for the *Wall Street Journal,* one in four Web visitors were "very concerned" and 49 percent were "somewhat concerned" about threats to their personal privacy on the Internet (Harris Interactive 2001). One in three Net users do not know what a "cookie" is, and more than 50 percent of Web respondents had never taken specific steps to protect their online privacy. Even simple protections, like monthly changes of passwords, are seldom done. Microsoft is introducing a high-tech solution, Platform for Privacy Preferences (P3P), to be installed in Version 6 of the company's Internet Explorer. Microsoft's P3P system would automatically interact with every web site as users surfed the Net, and consumers could decide whether to divulge any personal information based on P3P's rating of security at each site.

HIPAA PROVIDES PROTECTIONS

The Health Insurance Portability and Accountability Act of 1996 is the most extensive effort to regulate medical information and health-related transactions on the Internet. HIPAA does not just cover issues surrounding the Internet, but considers a wide range of electronic transactions wherever they occur, including electronic medical records, intranets, extranets, and private networks. A storm of controversy has been ignited over the 1,500 pages of small-print preamble and regulations to implement consumer privacy provisions of HIPAA, released in the December 28, 2000, issue of the *Federal Register* by the Health Care Financing Administration (HCFA). Preliminary federal regulations were originally released on October 29, 1999 and became final in December 2000 in the closing weeks of the Clinton administration. Release of the controversial rules came after a 15-month period for public comments and rule revisions. More than 52,000 comments were received, most from healthcare providers.

Upon taking over in 2001, Department of Health and Human Services Secretary Tommy Thompson of the new Bush administration promptly suspended implementation of HIPAA's privacy regulations and opened a second period for comment. Providers hope the new administration may scale back the new rules or extend the deadline for compliance. Industry groups ranging from the American Hospital Association to the American Association of Health Plans have strongly criticized the HIPAA regulations as prohibitively expensive to implement and disruptive to clinical operations (Tieman 2001a).

Some provisions of HIPAA are still being clarified by HCFA. Under the 1996 law, healthcare providers, health plans, and other third-party intermediaries will have two years, presumably until April 2003, to become compliant with privacy regulations. Related HIPAA regulations covering electronic transactions will go into effect in October 2002. However, some critics are calling for repeal of the extensive HIPAA regulations. Congressman Ron Paul, a physician, has submitted a House resolution to repeal the medical privacy rule (Snyder 2001).

PREPARING FOR HIPAA—THE NEXT Y2K

Coping with HIPAA will not be easy or cheap. Implementation will cost $17.6 billion, predicts HCFA, which would be offset by a projected $29.9 billion in savings over a ten-year period (DHHS Press Office 2000).

Providers, however, are skeptical of the government estimates. Information technology consultants predict that complying with HIPAA will take as much as or more than the work and costs of coping with Y2K (Howe 1999). A study for the American Hospital Association estimated HIPAA costs could be $22.5 billion over five years for hospitals, physicians, pharmacies, and insurance companies (Tieman and Bellandi 2001). One 400-bed hospital estimated its HIPAA costs at $2.5 million, about the same as Y2K (Heisey 2001).

Not everyone is complaining about HIPAA. At Minnesota's Allina Health System, a financial analysis by HIPAA program director Jeremy Pierotti shows a potential positive benefit of an additional $68 million to the system's cash flow from standardized electronic transactions, based on an $11 million investment and $79 million improvement in cash flow over a five-year period (Tieman 2001b). HIPAA is expected to simplify and consolidate the approximately 400 different electronic claims forms now in use into just a few uniform formats that everyone in the health industry would use, including doctors, hospitals, health plans, and patients.

Hospitals are already falling behind in addressing HIPAA. A recent survey of hospital operations and information systems managers by the Health Information and Management Systems Society (HIMSS) found that only 18 percent of hospitals have implemented policies and processes under HIPAA's new standards for security and confidentiality (Nelson Publishing 1999). Another survey of hospitals found that only one in three had a designated budget line for HIPAA compliance and remediation in 2001 (Heisey 2001). Healthcare IT analysts predict that most HIPAA spending will occur in 2002.

Complying with HIPAA has become the primary IT priority of American hospitals and health systems, according to the 12th Annual HIMSS Leadership Survey (HIMSS 2001). HIPAA compliance was cited by 79 percent of CIOS and healthcare information specialists in the survey, compared with 70 percent in 2000. Many hospitals and health systems are still ascending the HIPAA learning curve. Only 30 percent of healthcare information managers rated their organizations as "highly knowledgeable" about HIPAA, and just one in three institutions had hired a HIPAA compliance officer at the time of the survey, released in

February 2001. One in six (14 percent) hospitals had not even begun implementing compliance procedures. But progress has been made. An earlier national survey in April 1999, conducted by *Health Informatics Pulse* found that 60 percent of hospitals had not even begun to work on HIPAA compliance (AHIMA 1999).

Many providers have been waiting for HIPAA rules to become final before getting organized. The one in six healthcare organizations that have not started on HIPAA are at high risk of ending up handling their HIPAA transition in a crisis mode (Christianson 1999). Hospitals and physicians did not worry as much about electronic data transfer in the past, when few providers had installed electronic medical records. Security was less of an issue when many healthcare software packages and much computer hardware were incompatible from vendor to vendor. That is changing rapidly now, with intranets and extranets linking local providers into regional and national data networks. Healthcare information transfer is becoming "frictionless." The arrival of national, uniform standards is inevitable and long overdue.

The most important features of HIPAA relating to a provider's information technology system include the following (Browne 1999):

- Software systems must change to accommodate unique identifiers and standard transaction formats.
- Filing systems for submitting health insurance claims must change to include processes that support the claim filing.
- Software systems and electronic record-keeping systems must use specific coding and security standards.
- New policies and procedures are required for the electronic storage and maintenance of information.
- Users of individually identifiable healthcare information must meet measures of compliance in information security processes.

HIPAA EXPLAINED

For those unfamiliar with HIPAA, the primary purpose of this 1996 act is to guarantee health insurance access for consumers with prior health conditions (Aston 1999a). HIPAA is also known as the Kennedy-

Kassebaum bill, authored by Senator Nancy Kassebaum, who has since retired from the Senate. Key backers of HIPAA included Senators Edward Kennedy (D-Massachusetts) and Orin Hatch (R-Utah), whose bipartisan cosponsorship helped the bill become law. Standardizing electronic medical claims was a relatively minor administrative issue that was not addressed in detail in the legislation. Congress gave itself three years to develop and adopt implementation regulations, but the deadline for congressional action lapsed in mid-1999. The Clinton administration then released its own preliminary regulations on November 5, 1999, with a 60-day comment period—which stretched into 15 months in the face of extensive industry criticism. After their final release by the Clinton administration in December 2000, the HIPAA standards missed a deadline when HCFA regulators failed to send them to Congress for a 60-day review before final publication. Shortly thereafter, the Bush administration became involved, providing additional time for comments and opening the door for revisions. When the HIPAA rules are finalized, they will be self-implementing, with a deadline for compliance within 24 months after adoption, now slated for April 2003. Congress voted in an additional exemption for rural providers and small health plans, providing a third year for full compliance with HIPAA.

The arrival of Internet-enabled electronic commerce will be substantially facilitated when HIPAA is fully implemented. After years of frustration in the development of universal electronic standards, HIPAA represents a strong mandate from the federal government to automate health financial and clinical data. Under the terms of HIPAA, all major healthcare organizations must send electronic administrative information via electronic data interchange in a single standard. Electronic transmission of health data is a "tower of Babel" today, with over 400 different formats in use (Cupito 1999). In addition to providers, the law requires HMOs, health insurers, and other third-party administrators and clearinghouses to use a single HIPAA-defined administrative standard for electronic transactions such as claims and eligibility. Although the new rules will not eliminate paper transactions, sponsors hope that electronic data transmission will result in a simpler, lower-cost process.

The draft regulations promote a five-point program of consumer protection (DHHS 1999).

1. Consumer Control

Consumers are given important new rights, including the right to see a copy of their own medical records, to request a correction to their records, and to obtain documentation of any disclosures of their health information. Providers and health plans are required to educate patients on their HIPAA rights.

2. Boundaries on Medical Record Use and Release

An individual's health information can be used for health purposes only, including treatment, payment, and operations, and disclosures of information must be limited to the minimum necessary for the purpose of the disclosure. An exception is made for transfer of medical information for purposes of treatment, recognizing that physicians and other providers need access to the full patient record to provide quality care.

3. Security of Personal Health Information

Providers, health plans, and other organizations that handle medical information must establish written procedures to protect patients' privacy, designate a "privacy officer" to monitor the privacy program, and establish a grievance process for complaints about the privacy of their records.

4. Penalties

New penalty provisions are proposed for violations of a patient's right to privacy, with civil monetary penalties of $100 per incident, up to $25,000 per person, per year, per standard. Criminal penalties are also in place for certain kinds of privacy violations, with penalties up to $50,000 and one year in prison for disclosing or obtaining protected health information, and penalties up to $100,000 and five years in prison for obtaining health information under false pretenses. The biggest penalties—up to $250,000 in fines and ten years in prison—could be applied to anyone attempting to sell, transfer, use for commercial advantage, or cause personal gain or malicious harm.

5. Balancing Public Responsibility with Privacy Protections

HCFA specifically authorizes the routine disclosure of health information without individual authorization for a variety of activities that are of national interest and allow the health system to operate more smoothly. Special protection was also included for psychotherapy notes. These notes are held to a higher standard of protection, are not part of the medical record, and are never intended to be shared. Routine disclosures without authorization may be made for protected activities, such as:

- oversight of the healthcare system, including quality assurance;
- public health;
- research, assuming that a waiver of authorization has been approved by a privacy board or institutional review board;
- judicial and administrative proceedings;
- limited law enforcement activities;
- emergency circumstances;
- identification of the body of a deceased person or of the cause of death;
- facility patient directories; and
- activities related to national defense and security.

CONTROVERSY FOLLOWS CLINTON REGULATIONS FOR HIPAA

Four years after the release of HIPAA regulations, many aspects of its compliance are far from clear. Former DHHS Secretary Donna Shalala proposed new federal regulations for HIPAA in late October 1999, only months after Congress missed its August 1999 deadline to adopt rules to implement the act passed three years before. She was motivated by increasing consumer concerns that medical records were not nearly as private or secure as bank records or credit card transactions. Secretary Shalala had drafted a set of HIPAA recommendations and circulated them in September 1997, but the preliminary rules ran into a buzz saw of criticism from consumer groups and physicians regarding the lack of consumer privacy safeguards.

In a press conference in late October 1999, President Clinton praised the new draft of HIPAA regulations as protecting the "sanctity" of medical records (White House 1999). The President charged that the HIPAA regulations were intended to ensure that medical records did not "fall into the wrong hands." He noted that electronic records were already saving lives and reducing costs, but was concerned about the sense of vulnerability that many Americans feel about their medical records. He cited a poll in which two-thirds of consumers report they do not trust that their medical records will be kept safe.

The original draft regulations would impose a new set of uniform codes on all forms of electronic data transmission, but the new HIPAA regulations issued in December 2000 would cover data in any electronic format, as well as digitized paper records and oral communications. This sweeping expansion of the scope of regulations has drawn immediate criticism and could be eliminated if the Bush administration rewrites the HIPAA rules. The Clinton administration's December 2000 announcement of HIPAA regulations sparked new controversy, leading critics to complain that the administration had gone beyond the law in interpreting the legislation. Protests have centered on the provision in the final HIPAA regulations that call for providers and health plans to obtain specific patient consent for "routine disclosures" from health records, such as payment, treatment, healthcare operations, and internal data gathering. Hospitals and insurers have loudly protested this expansion of the regulations, but many physicians had commented to HCFA that advance consent should be obtained for such disclosures. Providers were also given general latitude to decide what "minimum" personal health information could be shared when sending medical records to other providers, after the breadth of the term "minimum information" had been questioned. The government has also specifically excluded access to patients' personal health information without authorization from the patient.

The goal of HIPAA is to establish national standards for electronic data transmission in healthcare, but the roles of states in regulating the Internet healthcare domain are not fully resolved. The federal government's HIPAA standards are clashing with regulations adopted by proactive states like New York that currently prohibit disclosing patient information or demographics on the Internet (*Computerworld* 1999). New Jersey has enacted state legislation that would require New Jersey health plans to be in HIPAA compliance within six months, and providers within one year. The New Jersey law has drawn a stiff counter-reaction and may be revised or rescinded. Secretary Donna Shalala's initial press release insisted that the draft HIPAA regulations would not limit or reduce other, stronger protections for confidentiality of health information, such as state legislation or regulations (DHHS 1999). The final rules published in December 2000 reaffirm that states could set stronger standards, which HIPAA would not pre-empt. The issue of conflicting state and federal standards could be a red flag for new DHHS Secretary Thompson, a former governor.

HIPAA'S IMPACT ON HEALTHCARE PROVIDERS

HIPAA could boost efficiency in the health sector. The health industry has lagged behind other sectors of the economy in automating data and electronic transactions. Despite the widespread adoption of computers in medicine and healthcare organizations, only an estimated 50 percent of all health claims are submitted electronically each year (Cupito 1999). Although hospitals and pharmacies submit a higher percentage of electronic claims, physician and dental claims lag behind. Faced with rising costs for submitting paper claims, virtually all providers and health plans will convert to full automation for electronic transactions within three to five years. In addition to transactions and coding standards, HIPAA will provide a unique electronic identification number for each of the 1.2 million provider entities today and issue another 30,000 to 40,000 electronic ID numbers each year in the future.

Cost savings are one of the major goals of HIPAA. Preliminary estimates by HCFA regulators show that providers would save $1.6 billion by the date of full compliance, currently set for 2003, and that health plans would also gain $1.6 billion in administrative efficiencies (Cupito 1999). Full savings from HIPAA will probably never be known because many providers and health plans are already moving rapidly to automate their e-commerce transactions and put them on the Internet. For health plans, third-parties, and clearinghouses, HIPAA will relieve them of scanning paper claims into the computer. The problem is complicated by many different forms used by various managed care plans, as well as by hard-to-read forms with tightly packed data that must be hand-entered. "Clean" electronic claims can be scanned, approved, and paid within seconds. Slow payment is a long-standing provider complaint, and many hospitals and doctors have experienced lengthy delays in getting paid by health plans.

HIPAA will be a powerful stimulus for automating medical records and electronic transactions in doctors' offices. Physician offices may be the least well prepared for HIPAA: Only one in four physicians are informed about HIPAA, according to a recent survey and many doctors appear to be unaware that HIPAA applies to their offices, not just hospitals and health plans. Larger medical groups may be in a better position to comply with HIPAA. Y2K has already spurred a number of physician offices to upgrade their data systems, allowing them to submit electronic claims. The high cost of information systems has also driven many physicians into group practice settings, which have the capital and expertise to manage large-scale data systems.

Some health plans have also lagged in the conversion to full electronic interchange, but Y2K accelerated their conversion from paper claims to automation in the past two years. Fear of Y2K glitches motivated every hospital and health plan in the United States to upgrade or fix equipment and software found to be noncompliant. As a result, very few providers or insurers experienced any Y2K mishaps in January 2000. The long-term impact of complying with HIPAA will reinforce the start made under Y2K—the creation of a national technology platform that is essentially universal between healthcare provider entities and health plans.

Hospitals and doctors will produce better, "cleaner" claims under HIPAA. The act reinforces federal efforts to standardize coding and claims. At the University of Wisconsin Hospital and Clinics in Madison, the finance department is delighted that HIPAA will standardize coding and eliminate an "archaic business process" in which the hospital now must pay clerical staff to input data from one computer to another (Sarudi 2001). For hospitals, the DRG methodology is stable and generally accepted, but physician billing is another matter. Physician coding under the evaluation and management (E&M) system is still a work in progress. Adopted in 1994, the E&M standards place significant new burdens on physicians to document their activities. Some physicians are voluntarily down coding and billing at a lower code than their services justify, out of fear of penalty. HIPAA will facilitate automated enforcement systems that will scan for patterns of errors or fraud by physicians.

HIPAA ATTACKS FRAUD AND ABUSE

Reduction of fraud and abuse in billings is another HIPAA goal. Relying on the False Claims Act, a Civil War–era law, the federal government will screen claims and back up allegations by whistle-blowers. Monetary penalties are triple the overcharged amount plus up to $10,000 per violation. In 1997, the federal government collected $1.2 million in civil settlements and recoveries. Full automation of electronic claims will allow payers like Medicare or Blue Cross to scan for patterns of abuse, such as faked auto injuries or disability requests. Pharmacy benefit management companies can be even more vigilant about overprescribing, as well as reducing medication errors. In Texas, an electronic detection system has been installed in the state's new automated Medicaid payment software. The goal is to recoup a projected $15 million in savings over a three-year period at a system upgrade cost of $5.7 million (Cupito 1999). EDS, based in Plano, Texas, is collaborating with Intelligent Technologies Corporation and HNC Software to create the new Medicaid fraud–busting system. Profiles for physicians, patients, and physician-patient partners will be developed and shared with the providers.

DEVELOPMENT OF HIPAA RULES

The lack of electronic standards and the compatibility concerns that HIPAA addresses are not new. For nearly a decade, healthcare providers and health plans have been working with government to standardize electronic data transmission in the health field. To expedite the transition to national standards, the Workgroup for Electronic Data Interchange (WEDI) was founded in 1991, with support from important provider organizations such as the American Medical Association (Aston 1999b). Today, WEDI has 130 corporate and individual members and an annual budget of $300,000. The group has no formal authority but has put the weight of its sponsors behind its efforts to prioritize and reach consensus on key issues surrounding electronic interchange. But hammering out agreements has been slow and complex. Another cooperating body is the Tunitas Group, a multisponsor health industry group that includes Kaiser Permanente, Catholic Healthcare West, and PacifiCare (*American Medical News* 1999).

Critics charge that the privacy rules are overdue and should be stricter. Janlori Goldman, director of Georgetown University's Health Privacy Project, states, "Everyone—Republicans, Democrats, all the advocacy groups—have said we need to limit this. Federal law is tougher on video-rental records than it is on protecting the privacy of patients' medical records" (Murray 1999, p. A3).

Everyone agrees that consumers' privacy should be respected in transmission of patients' fiscal, demographic, or clinical data. But federal standards for electronic privacy still lack definition, and developing data compliance programs may be difficult for providers without answers to issues like the following (Faulkner & Gray 1999):

- Who can, or should, get access to electronic medical records?
- What information is appropriate to be shared without a patient's permission?
- Under what circumstances should access to patient data be allowed or limited?

- What is the definition of an "agent" or a "trustee" of an organization responsible for ensuring electronic records privacy?
- What is the definition of "need to know"?
- What constitutes a "mistake" as opposed to willful disregard for the privacy laws?
- What authorization policies should be in place to ensure that a patient is not denied access?
- Which data elements (fields) should be required under the statute?

Not all HMOs and health plans are welcoming a standardization of electronic data transmissions. Some payers would rather continue to use their own claims and data formats, and a few plans have told the federal government they might pay fines for noncompliance rather than switch to national standards (Faulkner & Gray 1999). The costs to payers to implement HIPAA could reach billions of dollars. Hospitals and doctors report that their days in receivables has stretched to well over 75 days, and some providers wait more than 120 days for claims. Slow reimbursement allows the plans to gain interest revenues. The issue has soured relations with providers and stimulated "prompt payment" legislation to be enacted in many states.

HIPAA has created a firestorm of protest over various consumer provisions, such as the right to sue when privacy rights have been violated and a limit of $50,000 on such suits (Aston 1999b). Major controversy has also arisen regarding access to electronic medical records by law enforcement officials. Consumer groups and public-service law firms are linking with physicians and other providers to demand limits on access to patient data by law enforcement. Another problematic issue is access to medical data by juveniles, which some Republican representatives want HIPAA to respect under existing state laws. Health plans and business groups want HIPAA to preempt state regulations because the often-conflicting state rules increase administrative costs and limit efficiency. Some key Democrats are siding with consumer organizations and provider groups like the American Medical Association; they want to allow states to write patient privacy statutes, which would be even tougher than HIPAA. Dr. Thomas Reardon, president of the AMA, believes that, "patients won't be willing to share important health information with their doctors if they feel it could be disclosed inappropriately (Aston 1999b, p. 5).

PUBLIC-KEY INFRASTRUCTURE

The new federal HIPAA regulations are likely to drive healthcare organizations to adopt public-key infrastructure (PKI) within the next five years. PKI is the protocol used in digital certificates, a form of electronic identification that attests to the identity of a person or company before decrypting files (*Computerworld* 1999). In San Francisco, Catholic Healthcare West plans to use PKI to secure its e-mail, but in the interim is relying on nine regional data servers provided by WorldTalk in Santa Clara, California.

The three biggest problems facing providers who must develop PKI are (1) lack of data format and content standards, (2) cost of converting from paper-based to electronic systems, and (3) concerns about confidentiality of patient information.

EMRS AND CHINS

National standards for electronic medical records may be another by-product of HIPAA. Although federal law does not require standards for electronic medical records (EMRS), it does direct the National Committee on Vital and Health Statistics to study the issues related to uniform data standards for patient medical record information and the electronic transmission of such patient data. The standardization of medical records is sure to be opposed by thousands of vendors selling non-standard and proprietary EMRS today. The standardization of electronic medical records could make possible a national quality improvement program, as well as providing uniform data for report cards on provider and plan performance.

HIPAA could also revive the concept of community health information networks jointly shared by payers, providers, and purchasers. The CHIN concept of a shared hub-and-spoke model was proposed in the early 1990s, but it faltered under complexities of competing data requirements and formats. The problem from the beginning has been, "how do you fund and govern the thing?" (Christianson 1999). Who will voluntarily subsidize the costs of constructing and operating the CHINS? The first few CHINS were launched with foundation funding, but these pilots never evolved into a successful business model. Getting all the parties in an information exchange network to trust each other and give up information control is a daunting task. Standardizing healthcare's electronic transactions under HIPAA may make it possible for private or nonprofit CHIN entities to take on a clearinghouse function on a profitable, sustainable basis.

HIPAA CHECKLIST

Sandra Fuller of the American Health Information Management Association predicts that the overall goal of HIPAA is administrative simplification, but implementation within an organization will be anything but simple (Fuller 1999, p. 1). Few healthcare organizations across the nation have done much thinking or planning for HIPAA. The process of developing rules for HIPAA has taken so long, three years, that many providers have simply taken a wait-and-see attitude. Now the new rules for HIPAA are here, and most healthcare organizations and health plans will have only two years to become compliant. The health industry impact will be so widespread that some are calling it "the next Y2K" or even "Y2K on steroids" (Phoenix Health Systems 1999). By one estimate, healthcare providers will spend 33 percent of their information systems budgets on HIPAA for the next two years. Complying with HIPAA is not optional. JCAHO announced in the fall of 1999 that it would assess the security protections for information in every JCAHO-surveyed hospital or provider entity.

As the new millennium begins, the health industry has information tools that will potentially allow providers and health plans to achieve business goals at lightning speed (Browne 1999, p. 54). But as the pace of healthcare's information technology deployment increases, the issue of patient privacy lags behind. To jump-start the transition, the American Health Information Management Association has developed a

HIPAA checklist that every provider organization can use as it prepares for HIPAA (see Figure 11.1). The HIPAA requirements are complex, and many provisions will need additional clarification from the federal Department of Health and Human Services.

CONSULTING FIRMS ORGANIZE FOR HIPAA

Feeling overwhelmed by HIPAA? Help can be on the way, at a price. Information technology consulting firms are already gearing up to assist clients in HIPAA compliance, including initial HIPAA readiness assessment, work plan creation to achieve HIPAA certification, standardization of policies and procedures, and recommendations for management structures to direct all HIPAA compliance activities. The costs and complexity of becoming HIPAA compliant are likely to accelerate the outsourcing of information systems management to experienced healthcare IT consulting firms.

The budget of a HIPAA consulting project can range from $196,500 for a single hospital to $570,000 for a multihospital system using a hypothetical cost estimate. As a practical matter, some hospitals and systems may be able to manage their HIPAA review and compliance with less outside assistance, and others may lack the staffing, in-house expertise, or time as the HIPAA deadline nears and thus be compelled to rely on consultants more heavily.

Two years may be barely enough to meet the challenge of becoming HIPAA compliant. Most providers have only a superficial understanding of how time consuming and resource intensive this upgrading process may be (AHIMA 1999). In Salinas, California, the Salinas Valley Memorial Healthcare System began preparing for HIPAA in 1997. The health system's IT director, Tom Duncan, and Suad Picardi, computer systems security analyst, estimate they spend 15 to 20 percent of their time on HIPAA-related issues and preparation, at an annual cost of $50,000. For Salinas, education was the first-priority strategy. The hospital operates medical and health facilities in 52 sites, so the payoff will be not only HIPAA compliance, but a working knowledge of information security practices by all managers, employees, and medical staff.

Figure 11.1: HIPAA Checklist

The AHIMA checklist is an excellent place to begin the organizational assessment, which is the first step in obtaining HIPAA compliance certification (Fuller 1999)

1. Getting Organized

    1.1 Assign responsibility for tracking the progress of regulations during the comment period
    1.2 Inform key stakeholders about HIPAA, e.g., board, medical staff executive committee, senior management team
    1.3 Identify HIPAA's impending impact on the organization's information systems and processes
    1.4 Seek current information from expert organizations and consultants on HIPAA compliance
    1.5 Prepare a communications plan for implementation of HIPAA, e.g., publications, seminars, web sites
    1.6 Conduct educational programs to orient administrative and clinical leaders about HIPAA requirements, e.g., nursing staff, medical staff

2. Standardization of Code Sets

    2.1 Monitor payer compliance with official coding guidelines
    2.2 Perform regular coding quality control studies
    2.3 Provide feedback on documentation issues that affect the quality of coded data
    2.4 Routinely train coding staff on current coding practices
    2.5 Provide access to resources available on coding guidelines and best practices
    2.6 Efficiently update the codes for ICD-9-CM and CPT-4

3. Healthcare Identifiers

    3.1 Assess the quality of the master person index (MPI)
    3.2 Perform required clean-up of the MPI
    3.3 Institute procedures to maintain the integrity of the MPI
    3.4 Train staff on the importance of data quality in an MPI

continued on following page

Figure 11.1 *(continued from previous page)*

3.5 Make necessary data quality improvements in the registration systems
3.6 Create an enterprisewide MPI
3.7 Eliminate duplications in the enterprisewide MPI
3.8 Assign responsibility for maintenance of MPI data integrity

4. Provider Database

4.1 Perform routine data integrity checks on the provider database
4.2 Develop effective procedures to maintain provider tables
4.3 Integrate or interface provider tables to necessary systems
4.4 Monitor data quality for unique personal identification numbers (UPINS) on billing documents
4.5 Provide easy access to UPIN tables

5. Payer Linkages

5.1 Maintain complete payer tables
5.2 Perform data quality checks on payer data entry
5.3 Develop feedback loops from the billing process to data collection processes regarding payer data

6. Claims Transactions

6.1 Maintain effective communication regarding claims processing with all affected parties
6.2 Perform routine maintenance on the charge master
6.3 Utilize electronic claims processing and electronic data interchange
6.4 Explore feasibility of converting to electronic claims processing or outsourcing the function
6.5 Have comprehensive documentation of claims processing
6.6 Perform routine monitor remittance information against claims data
6.7 Have an effective process for handling rejected claims
6.8 Aggregate data about rejected claims to improve claims processing
6.9 Become familiar with the transaction rules of standards-setting organizations

continued on following page

Figure 11.1 *(continued from previous page)*

7. Information Security

    7.1   Ensure that organizational structures exist to develop and implement an information security program

    7.2   Implement policies to control access to and release of patient-identifiable health information

    7.3   Ensure that users of electronic health information have unique access codes

    7.4   Ensure that each user's access is restricted to the information needed to do his or her job

    7.5   Ensure that medical staff bylaws, rules, and regulations outline physician responsibilities for protecting the confidentiality of health information

    7.6   Employee handbook must outline employee responsibilities for protecting confidentiality of health information

    7.7   Everyone with access to health information must receive specific training about confidentiality and responsibilities

    7.8   Ensure that all vendor contracts for outsourcing health information functions include provisions regarding confidentiality and information security

    7.9   Information system managers, network managers, and programmers must not have unlimited or unrecorded access to patient information

    7.10   Ensure that monitor access to information and corrective action plans are in place for violation of organization policy

    7.11   Perform risk assessments that are utilized to prioritize and continually improve the security of the systems

    7.12   Ensure current knowledge of information security issues and industry responses by providing informational resources, such as books, publications, seminars

Source: Adapted from Fuller (1999).

Health systems with multiple hospitals can leverage their HIPAA knowledge across several locations, but HIPAA conformance can be more complex when not all hospitals operate with the same set of information technologies and software systems. In Oregon, the hospitals of the Providence Health System launched their HIPAA initiative in January 2000, as soon as they had put Y2K in the rear-view mirror (Sarudi 2001). They organized a large multidisciplinary committee of nearly 30, including practicing physicians. The system's "gap analysis" of 14 cost centers included hiring an information security consultant to try to break through the network's firewalls, and an attorney to review Providence's policies and procedures. The Providence system found few significant lapses, although in one case, paper in blue bins intended for recycling as scratch pads turned out to have confidential patient information. Providence is now rewriting policies and processes and expects to complete its HIPAA remediation by January 2002.

HIPAA certification will require providers, plans, and third parties to attend to the following issues (Fuller 1999).

Security Management Process. Begin the HIPAA compliance process by designating someone within the organization as responsible for managing the HIPAA security process. This function will involve risk analysis, risk management, security policy, and sanctions.

Applications and Data Criticality Analysis. The process of Y2K readiness will be helpful as health organizations begin an inventory of information systems. The management team handling HIPAA compliance must determine whether the systems and data are critical to patient care or central to the organization's business. All IT system reviews must be carefully documented. Systems and data should then be categorized by priority.

Data Backup Plan. Organizations must develop a written policy that outlines how data will be backed up, addressing the issues of how often, how complete, who performs, who is responsible, where the data are stored, and where the data are tested.

Emergency Mode Plan. The organization must develop procedures for data operations in case of an emergency, including assessment of power alternatives, hardware alternatives, "hot site" alternatives, and manual alternatives.

Testing and Revision Procedures. Software must be tested to ensure the organization's data integrity. The testing should include version controls, data conversions, and data safeguards.

Processing Records. Appoint someone to be responsible for processing medical records. Establish procedures for processing EMRS, focusing on receipt, manipulation, storage, dissemination, transmission, and disposal.

Access Control. Under HIPAA, only certain people are allowed access to an organization's data and medical records. The organization must establish a process to determine how authorization will be established and modified. Develop an "access grid," which outlines employees' duties as they are connected to data access. As an employee's duties change, so must the grid. If an employee is terminated, access must be revoked immediately. This process must be carefully documented.

Internal Audit Process. One key individual should be designated as responsible for the internal audit of data and systems. The internal audit function includes process and policy development, technical enhancements, and disciplinary action relating to data access.

Personnel Security. Issues of HIPAA personnel security involve supervision, maintenance of access records, clearance, and training. Personnel policies must be revised or expanded as necessary to incorporate new HIPAA-compliance processes. All polices and processes must be adequately documented.

System Configuration Management. As hospitals and health systems develop regional and national networks, the HIPAA security protocols and processes must extend across all participants in the network.

Security Incident Procedures. If and when data security lapses occur, the organization must have a process for reporting and addressing them. The security incident process must answer questions such as the following: Who collects the information? Who is responsible for reporting the information? What events are reportable? What is the response?

Media Controls. This procedure covers the receipt and removal of hardware, software, and data from the system when necessary.

Physical Access. This process outlines when the following would go into effect: disaster recovery, emergency operations, equipment control, facility security plan, maintenance records, need-to-know procedures, sign-in, testing, and revision.

Workstation Use. Outline the proper functions for automatic logoff, screen position, sign-on, and sign-off.

THE STRUGGLE TO IMPLEMENT HIPAA

Health systems and larger hospitals can piggy-back HIPAA with their in-place compliance program for Medicare fraud and abuse. Larger providers have established operational compliance programs, which can be used as a baseline for developing HIPAA-certified systems. They may be able to utilize compliance processes and staff as the working infrastructure for HIPAA compliance. But smaller hospitals and medical groups do not have the same resources as larger facilities and health systems. HIPAA may require substantial investments in information technology. Providers now operating on slim margins may face real difficulties with the need for more IT capital expenditures (Christianson 1999).

Doctors in solo practices and small groups will probably find HIPAA overwhelming. The federal government recommends that doctors work with a consultant to implement the HIPAA security requirements. Small medical groups will be given an additional year (three total) to comply with HIPAA. Even small medical offices must provide or implement the following (Gomolski 1999):

* evaluation by a consultant or practice management system vendor;

- personnel security policies;
- assigned security responsibility (the "HIPAA officer");
- compliant hardware;
- software with internal audit trail capability;
- facilities requirements, such as rooms or closets with locks to safeguard equipment;
- employee training;
- chain-of-trust agreements with claims processors; and
- documentation that is maintained and updated.

Providers, health plans, and suppliers must act quickly to accommodate HIPAA, but most organizations will have at least two years to become compliant, and Congress may extend the deadline. Smaller and rural providers already get a third year to gain HIPAA certification. Market analysts predict that most HIPAA-compliance work will occur in 2002, after the regulations have stabilized. This will allow time for consulting firms and early compliers to test their HIPAA methodologies. Federal regulators will also need time to design standard tests for HIPAA compliance. Given the controversy about releasing HIPAA regulations during the transition of presidential administrations, Congress may not allow all parties another two to three years to organize for HIPAA.

LOOKING FORWARD: HIPAA IS AN OPPORTUNITY

Suppliers, service bureaus, and consulting firms should be part of the strategic IT planning process to address HIPAA successfully. Consider them partners as well as vendors. These outside organizations can provide expertise, assessment, action recommendations, and ready-to-install systems, which can be customized to each provider entity. First-movers in the market who respond to HIPAA can become beta sites to test new programs, a process which can reduce fees and even capital costs during the evaluation process. Once HIPAA's national standards and processes are put into place, the economic savings achieved by reducing administrative expenses can be substantial. HIPAA today is a speed-bump on the information highway, but in the future, HIPAA compliance will be a launching ramp for the long-awaited implementation of universal electronic transactions in the health field.

STRATEGIC IMPLICATIONS

Implementing HIPAA will be costly and complicated, but there is a silver lining. Pulling health-related IS and IT out of the post-Y2K doldrums, HIPAA will reignite the momentum toward the digital transformation of American healthcare.

Reassess IT Needs and Systems. Use HIPAA as an opportunity to reassess current information technology needs and systems. Conduct an e-health audit to identify all the Internet connections, Web-enabled business functions, and future linkages with doctors, payers, suppliers, and other partners.

Update Strategies. Update the organization's information systems strategies, information-supported functions, and capital investment plans for information technology. HIPAA allows an opportunity to reassess relationships with health plans and suppliers. Create strategic partnerships to share best practices, consultants, and costs.

Consolidate Compliance and HIPAA. Some healthcare provider organizations may want to consolidate their compliance programs and designate the chief information officer as the responsible official for HIPAA as well as for Medicare compliance.

Remember the Human Factor. HIPAA is not just about upgrading information technology and rewriting policies. Training employees, nurses, and physicians how to handle sensitive patient information is the capstone of ensuring security and confidentiality for patients.

REFERENCES

American Health Information Management Association (AHIMA). 1999. "Leading the Way to HIPAA Security Requirements." Briefing memo for members, August, pp. 1–3.

American Medical News. 1999. "Tunitas Group Formed to Facilitate Electronic Transactions." *American Medical News* 42 (28): 5.

Aston, G. 1999a. "Health Insurance Law Falling Short." [Online news article.] *American Medical News,* March 15, pp. 1–3.

———. 1999b. "Work on Privacy Bill Continues." *American Medical News* 42 (34): 5.

Browne, D. 1999. "Patient Privacy Issues Facing Health Care." *Houston Business Journal* 30 (23): 54A.

Computerworld. 1999. "Digital Protection for Health Care E-Mail Seeks to Standardize Electronic Transmission." [Online news report.] *Computerworld,* March 1, pp. 1–2.

Christianson, J. 1999. "HIPAA Update Midyear 1999: A Review of a Seminar by Lee Barrett." Internal memorandum (unpublished), July 14, pp. 1–2. Southfield, MI: Superior Consultant.

Cupito. M. C. 1999. "Paper Cuts? HIPAA's New Rules Pushed for Electronic Commerce Within Healthcare Industry." *Health Management Technology* 19 (8): 34–35.

Department of Health and Human Services (DHHS). 1999. "HHS Proposes First-Ever National Standards to Protect Patients' Personal Medical Records." Press release, October 29, pp. 1–4. Washington, DC: DHHS.

Department of Health and Human Services (DHHS) Press Office. 2000. *Protecting the Privacy of Patients' Health Information, Summary of the Final Regulation,* December 20, pp. 1–5. Washington, DC: DHHS.

Faulkner & Gray. 1999. "HIPAA Could Spur Transactions." Cited in internal memorandum, December 17, p. 1. Southfield, MI: Superior Consultant.

Fried, B. M. 2001. "Regulating the E-Health Industry." *Medicine on the Net* 7 (3): 7–8.

Fuller, S. 1999. "HIPAA Checklist." Special report, American Health Information Management Association.

Gomolski, B. C. 1999. "Hospitals Face Info Overhauls." [Online news story.] *Computerworld* 32 (21): 39.

Harris Interactive. 2001. "Exposure in Cyber-Space." [Online survey.] *Wall Street Journal,* March 21, p. B1.

Heisey, L. 2001. "HIPAA and Healthcare IT." *Off-the-Record Research,* February, pp. 1–5.

Health Information Management Systems Society (HIMSS). 2001. "HIPAA Displaces Internet Technologies as Top Priorities for IT Organizations." Press release, February 5, pp. 1–5. Chicago: HIMSS.

Howe, R. 1999. "HIPAA: Overview of New Federal Regulations." PowerPoint presentation, November. Southfield, MI: Superior Consultant.

Murray. S. 1999. "Clinton Seeks Compromise on Medical Records." *Wall Street Journal,* October 25, p. A3.

Nelson Publishing. 1999. "Slow Progress in Healthcare HIPAA Data Security Standards Compliance." [Online news summary.] *Health Management Technology* 20 (19): 6.

Phoenix Health Systems. 1999. "What to Expect from HIPAA." [Online newsletter.] *HIPPALERT* 1 (1): 1–5.

Poulsen, K. 2000. "Hospital Records Hacked." [Online news story.] December 6, pp. 1–3.

Sarudi, D. 2001. "HIPAA Early Adopters." *Hospitals & Health Networks* 75 (2): 38–44.

Simpson, G. R. 2001. "The Battle over Web Privacy." *Wall Street Journal,* March 21, pp. B1, B4.

Snyder, K. 2001. "Alert: Medical Privacy." [Online news release.] *The Liberty Activist,* March 15, pp. 1–2.

Tieman, J. 2001a. "A Second Chance: New Public Comment Period Gives Industry a Shot at Reining in HIPAA." *Modern Healthcare* 31 (10): 14.

———. 2001b. "Praise HIPAA: Some Providers Embrace Privacy Regulations in Hopes of Securing Long-Term Savings." *Modern Healthcare* 31 (13): 36–40.

Tieman, J., and D. Bellandi. 2001. "HIPAA Will Be No Holiday." *Modern Healthcare* 31 (1): 3, 15.

White House. 1999. "Remarks by the President on Medical Privacy in the Oval Office," October 29, pp. 1–3. Washington, DC: Office of the Press Secretary.

Wall Street Journal. 2001. "Privacy vs. Productivity: A Tough Choice." *Wall Street Journal,* March 8, p. A1.

wsj.com. 2001. "Industry Groups Launch Attack on Internet-Privacy Legislation." [Online news story.] *Wall Street Journal,* March 13, p. 1.

CHAPTER TWELVE

Managing Healthcare's E-Organizations

KEY CONCEPTS: Hard-wired, soft-wired •
Deconstructed • C-commerce • Digital hospital •
Knowledge management • E-reengineering • E-culture

INTRODUCTION: Healthcare organizations will never be the same in the post-information era. The management vision of the New Economy is that e-organizations will be "deconstructed," with flexible teams that design their own work, replacing large hierarchies of workers with well-defined jobs and tasks. In fact, the world of work has been changing long before "e" became a symbol for the information-enabled economy. "Collaborative commerce" is used to describe strategies that link a number of organizations into mutually supportive business relationships. Collaboration has the potential to transform a supply chain beyond simple transactions into true inter-enterprise partnerships. E-organizations are applying information technology and the Internet to transform the workplace and increase productivity. The new field of knowledge management provides customized workspaces that contain information, applications, and links specific to the functions of an individual, as well as the people-to-people communications needs of a work group. As the digital transformation occurs within the health sector, every hospital, medical group, health plan, and supplier must face the "e-culture challenge" to prepare themselves for the move to an e-based set of internal processes and external relationships.

"The hard-wired structure of the conventional corporate organization reflects the high cost of establishing information channels.

But as these costs fall, the organization can become 'soft-wired.' People can group and regroup into teams. Individuals can participate in multiple projects simultaneously. Teams in turn can team. Organization becomes continuously self-organizing and adapting .... The organization builds competitive advantage not from what it is or does, but from how it reviews, learns from, and then amends its own procedures and structure."

—*Philip Evans and Thomas Wurster (2000, p. 217)*

Underneath the hype and the hope for the electronic revolution is a real truth—organizations will never be the same in the post-information era. The management vision of the new economy is that e-organizations will be "deconstructed," with flexible teams that design their own work, replacing large hierarchies of workers with well-defined jobs and tasks. Futurist Jeff Goldsmith advises hospital executives to view the Web and Internet applications as a "rich and diverse toolbox for restructuring their relationships with their customers and reducing the cost of resolving their health problems" (Goldsmith 2001, p. 16).

After the decline of the dot-com market and an economic downturn labeled the "Internet recession," many companies are looking for the right mix of old-economy management methods and new-economy technology applications (Schwartz 2001). America's healthcare executives are turning to information technology and the Internet for applications that are "less glitzy but more apt to pay off where it counts: improvement of basic business capabilities in the face of continuing financial pressures," according to *Modern Healthcare's* annual survey of information system trends (Morrisey 2001). Capital expenditures for IT are starting to rise after the post-Y2K slump (see Figure 12.1). Hospitals plan to spend 8 percent more on new information technology next year, up from 7 percent in 2000 but well below the increases of 9.5 to 11 percent as hospitals geared up for Y2K between 1995 and 1998. Hospitals are holding down spending on information technology to 2.5 percent of operating budgets, off slightly from 2.6 percent last year.

Figure 12.1: Information Systems Priorities into 2003

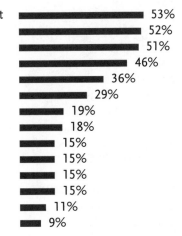

Use emerging technologies, e.g., Internet	53%
Address changes in JCAHO, HIPAA	52%
Improve decision support for clinicians	51%
Improve productivity and reduce costs	46%
Improve patient-care capabilities	36%
Integrate databases	29%
Improve patient-accounting abilities	19%
Tie cost of care to outcomes	18%
Use LANS	15%
Respond to consumer needs for info	15%
Prove benefit of technology	15%
Improve ambulatory capabilities	15%
Improve general accounting/payroll	11%
Improve managed care capabilities	9%

Source: Morrisey (2001).

Despite barriers to e-business, the healthcare industry is facing pressures from consumers, insurance carriers, and government to become electronically connected. CSC, a national information technology firm, recently conducted its Critical Issues of Information Systems study (Reeder 2001). This annual study, the 13th published by the *Healthcare Leadership & Management Report,* found that healthcare lagged behind most other industries in developing the connectivity for electronic-based business. Only 38 percent of healthcare organizations have an e-business strategy, but that trend is shifting upward. More patients are arriving in physicians' offices with online research about their conditions. They want online access to their medical records and claims and want to be able to e-mail their physicians and make appointments electronically. Physicians want similar access regarding authorizations, claims, and payments from managed care organizations, and government is pressuring providers to use electronic solutions to reduce medical errors. The CSC study concludes that healthcare executives "recognize the need to embrace e-technologies, but, for the most part, have yet to do so" (Reeder 2001, p. 24).

Table 12.1: Hospitals and Health Systems Rated Among the 100 Most Wired

Hospital/System	Total Employees	Clinical Retrieval	Supplier Functions	Payer Activities
Ancillla Systems	3,730	81–100%	1–20%	1–20%
Baylor University Medical Center	5,395	81–100	81–100	81–100
Henry Ford Health System	16,000	81–100	41–60	41–60
Lancaster Health Alliance*	5,000	41–60	81–100	21–40
Methodist Health System	8,837	61–80	81–100	81–100
Sentara HealthCare*	13,932	61–80	1–20	21–40
UPMC Health System*	29,000	61–80	1–20	61–80
University of Texas/MD Anderson	8,730	61–80	41–60	1–20
William Beaumont Hospital*	11,344	41–60	41–60	61–80
Yale–New Haven Hospital	8,143	81–100	21–40	41–60

*Also rated as one of the top 100 hospitals in the United States by Solucient.

Source: Solovy (2000).

BECOMING WIRED FOR THE NEW ECONOMY

Across the United States, the 100 most-wired hospitals and health systems are breaking new ground, demonstrating the potential of e-organizations. According to the annual survey for *Hospitals & Health Networks,* a growing e-commerce gap is emerging between the most wired and the rest of the nation's hospitals (Solovy 2000). The 100 most-wired institutions submit more claims online, automate more of their supply chain, and provide more clinical data to their patients. Four of the 100 most wired are also among the Solucient top 100–ranked hospitals in the United States (see Table 12.1).

The gap between the e-leaders and the rest of the healthcare industry is growing. The average hospital employs the Internet for 20 percent of its payer activities, versus 41 to 60 percent for the most wired. Hospitals and health systems rated among the top 100 e-organizations accomplish 33 percent of their eligibility verification and 22 percent of their precertification online, more than twice the rate of the typical hospital. The most wired achieve a significant return on investment from their e-strategies by reducing their costs on labor-intensive activities such as electronic claims and payment.

CONNECTIVITY, PRIVATE INTRANETS, AND C-COMMERCE

The technology to link software, hardware, and telecommunications solutions is rapidly becoming available at very affordable costs. Intranets and wireless communications link networks of PC-based workstations, handheld PDA-type electronic charts, and other devices such as medication scanners or telemonitors. Healthcare providers are gaining the ability to synchronize data from a Web-based intranet with the latest versions of Microsoft Outlook and Palm-type handheld devices (PR *Newswire* 2000). The concept of private intranets originated from idealab!, a Woburn, Massachusetts–based business incubator that has launched more than 50 Internet businesses since 1996. A growing number of hospitals are installing intranets to connect their medical staff with the hospital's data systems. Private intranet networks were among the top ten priorities of healthcare executives, according to *Modern Healthcare*'s annual survey (Morrisey 2001).

Innovative applications of electronic technology are flooding into the health field. In Illinois, the Sherman Hospital is partnering with Medi-Transport, an Elgin, Illinois–based ambulance firm, to install digital video cameras for transmitting images back to the hospital's emergency department (Health Care Advisory Board Daily Briefing 2001). The project is unique because it will transmit live video stream, not just still pictures. The digital video camera can shoot pictures at accident scenes as well as during treatment of patients en route to the emergency room.

"Collaborative commerce," or "c-commerce," is the term used to describe strategies that link a number of organizations into mutually supportive business relationships. According to *Gartner's Business Technology Journal,* c-commerce extends the concept of electronic business transactions into a trading community (Gartner 2000). Collaboration has the potential to transform a supply chain beyond simple transactions into true inter-enterprise partnerships. In a collaborative mode, partners can share data around functions like production planning, demand forecasting, and sales strategies. This can reduce costs, improve time to market, and provide insights into customer needs. By leveraging the partners' market reputations in a collaborative market approach, they can widen the sphere of current and potential customers.

The ability to share data and information in a collaborative manner provides a low-cost, wide-access infrastructure for pursuing mutual business goals. In Birmingham, Alabama, HealthSouth and Oracle have announced a joint venture to build a "digital hospital" that would be a model of information technology (*Wall Street Journal* 2001). Oracle chairman Larry Ellison, one of Silicon Valley's best-known CEOS, and HealthSouth chair Richard Scrushy are joining together to build, from the ground up, a hospital that closely integrates information technology with patient care. The new facility will have the latest automated systems, electronic medical records, and e-enabled quality-improvement programs with remote physician access to electronic records from any location.

HEALTHCARE APPLICATIONS OF TECHNOLOGY

Healthcare organizations are looking for the killer applications of information technology that will slash costs, improve outcomes, and send patients home more satisfied. The focus of IT investment is shifting from financial systems to clinical systems. A growing number of pioneering hospitals and health systems are implementing electronic medical records and electronic physician order entry (POE), including InterMountain Healthcare, the Mayo Clinic, Peace Health, University of Nebraska, and San Diego's Sharp HealthCare. The Montefiore Medical Center in New York has nearly 600 beds equipped with EMR and POE, which have helped reduce the incidence of medical errors by more than 50 percent (Byrne 2001).

Automated medications distribution systems are also a promising application of electronic technology to the problem of medical errors. Systems developed by vendors such as Bridge Medical of San Diego and the NextRx Corporation rely on bar-coded, prepackaged medications and computer-assisted dispensing systems to attack the problem of a 1 to 3 percent medication error rate in many U.S. hospitals (Mucklo 2001). Pharmaceuticals are sorted, dispensed, and verified by a high-tech drug packaging system in response to physician orders transmitted electronically to the pharmacy. Medications are loaded into a dispensing cart, which is wheeled from patient to patient on nursing floors. Bar codes on the medication packets are double-checked against bar codes on patients' wristband IDs. A handheld computer scanner tracks medications, dosages, time of administration, and drug incompatibilities. Wireless communications ensure that all medications are checked with doctors' orders.

E-technology can also assist with the problem of errors in diagnosis. For example, misinterpretation of mammogram results can lead to missed diagnoses of breast cancers; however, this can be prevented using a remarkable new digital imaging application of medical artificial intelligence developed by R2 Technology of Los Altos, California (Becker 2001). The company has introduced a computerized second reading of standard mammograms, which can improve an radiologist's accuracy by as much as 20 percent. Two years ago, the Food and Drug Administration approved the "Image Checker," a computer-assisted detection (CAD) system for mammography. Under new Congressional authorization in January 2001, Medicare will now pay $15 for the computer-assisted second reading, with the goal of cutting the 15 percent current rate of missed diagnoses by half.

INTERNET CUSTOMERS AND COMPETITORS

Every business today has Internet customers and Internet competitors. The most sought-after customers are the early Internet adopters, predicts the Institute of Management Administration (IOMA 2000). They have a high degree of discretionary spending and expect high-quality customer service. The companies that succeed will have taken both offensive and defensive options, from reinventing their core customer strategies to exiting their current business before it has been commoditized by other Internet-based competitors. In the computer field, Compaq has followed the lead of Dell, letting customers design their own computers online and getting them built to order. IBM could not compete with Dell in the PC market, and thus exited. Higher education is another field feeling the impact of the Internet. A recent survey by InterEd reported that 75 percent of universities will offer online coursework, sell texts and books online, and conduct online seminars in the future (McGowan 2000).

Competitive strategy in the health field is being challenged by new Internet-based options. Health benefit management consultants like Hewitt and Wyatt Worldwide are developing electronic options for their employer customers. The alternative is to risk losing them to e-competitors like HealthAxis and eHealthInsurance.com. Healthcare professional organizations are confronting e-based challenges, from online news services to distance-learning providers. At the American Society of Association Executives in Silver Spring, Maryland, association executives are recognizing that the Web "was challenging our assumptions about who we were, what we do, and how we do it" (Eisinger 2000). The Internet is a direct competitor to most associations' reliance on their annual meetings, as suppliers develop new channels to association members. Associations are responding by developing interactive web sites, online discussion groups, distance-learning programs, and online news services to rebuild the loyalty of their members and offer new electronic product lines to replace lost revenues.

EXPEDITING THE PROCESSES OF CHANGE AND KNOWLEDGE MANAGEMENT

Business management students are learning how to use an electronic toolkit to accelerate the process of organizational change. A new set of business decision-support software called the "Matrix of Change," developed by Base-Six, a Boston-based business development consulting firm, is teaching students at Massachusetts Institute of Technology Sloan School of Management and other leading business schools how to identify the organizational capital in an enterprise (*Internet Wire* 2001). Organizational capital is often ten times more valuable than the technology capital deployed within a company. The software focuses analysis on six key organizational functions, including strategy, marketing, branding, user experience, technology, and program management.

IBM is one of many companies involved in assisting organizations to make more effective use of their employees' valuable knowledge. The field of knowledge management will rapidly expand in the next five years, growing 43 percent to $4.8 billion by 2004, according to IDC, a market research firm (Barger 2000). IBM's latest offering in the field of knowledge management is customized workspaces that contain information, applications, and links specific to the functions of an individual, as well as the people-to-people communications needs of a work group.

ENTERING AN E-PARTNERSHIP

Many hospitals and health systems find themselves partnering with new-economy companies in electronic-based businesses that offer web site hosting, intranet development, supply-chain management, electronic medical records, wireless networks, and management of their information systems. Creating and managing strategic business partnerships is one of the hallmarks of successful e-organizations.

The "e" entered the healthcare environment almost five years ago, and a number of lessons are still to be learned about managing relationships with electronic enterprises. (Flory 2001).

- Overcoming lack of expertise: Use consultants to overcome a frequent hurdle for provider organizations entering e-business— lack of experience and expertise.
- Defining goals, priorities, and timetables: For new e-business relationships, define a sequence of goals and priorities to be accomplished over several phases. Setting measurable targets is essential for monitoring progress.
- Delineating partner selection criteria: Identify key criteria for comparing e-partners, specifying ideal and essential qualifications and experience and weighting the criteria.

- Selecting partners fairly and effectively: Develop a well-executed e-partner selection strategy and employ a decision process that includes a mix of managers and end users.
- Articulating decision factors and deal breakers: Tell potential e-partners what is most important, defining baseline criteria for performance. Clarification of key factors at the outset is the best way to get an e-partnering relationship off on the right footing.
- Forging an agreement based on more than money: Ensure alignment of the long-range goals and values of all participants.
- Investing in the relationship: A joint venture will either succeed or fail not only because of financial performance but because of the ability or inability of all parties to create a unified team culture.
- Making progress from the beginning: As early as possible, begin to deliver value from the e-business relationship to internal and external customers. Make services available on a trial basis, and modify them frequently based on user feedback. Overcome skepticism by delivering tangible outcomes on an incremental basis.
- Reflecting on progress: Meet frequently with the e-business partner to review progress and make joint decisions. Develop an interactive process that monitors implementation and adjusts plans continuously.
- Planning for the long-term: Injecting a new-economy business model and technology into healthcare's traditional old-economy mind-set cannot be done overnight.

DIGITAL STRATEGIES FOR HEALTHCARE ORGANIZATIONS

Healthcare executives have been advised in this book to outsource non-core-competency functions; focus on the key attributes of their business strategy; automate their supply chain; migrate to the Web at Internet speed; and transform as many operational, supplier, and customer-relations functions as possible. In these days of electronic globalization of markets and technological change at interplanetary speed, many healthcare executives are e-skeptics. They watch as the market for

Internet-based stock crashes and believe that e-hype has far exceeded any reasonable prospect of profit from electronic business strategies.

Skepticism is healthy in the short term, but when considering the long-range future, healthcare organizations must face the likelihood that "e" is not just another fad but that, in fact, the digital transformation of healthcare is a long-term trend for the new millennium. This technology meets the three most important criteria for market competition—it is better, faster, and cheaper (Coile 1999). In the future, every health executive, physician, and nurse will have at least one handheld personal digital assistant, will communicate on the Internet, and will never have to be out of touch because of 24 x 7 connectivity.

The electronic revolution is one of the fundamental market forces of the twenty-first century. No organization can ignore this megatrend; indeed, every healthcare executive should now ask, "What works?" and "Where is the return on investment" in the e-future. Because investment in IT typically absorbs at least 50 percent of capital projects by hospitals and health systems, healthcare executives are naturally concerned about return on investment. In Minneapolis, HealthSystem Minnesota is concerned that the organization needs to automate many of its clinical and administrative tasks but lacks the resources to do it. Their CIO admits, "As a $500 million organization, we aren't big enough to develop the IT systems we need. We can't get where we need to go if we do it incrementally. Therefore, we need a private firm as a capital partner (Coddington, Ackerman, and Moore 2001, p. 3).

Following are some preliminary lessons from the digital transition of other sectors of the economy, as well as early results from healthcare pioneers who are testing electronic solutions.

Financial Performance

Improving financial performance will be a major driver of the digital transformation of American healthcare. In 1996, hospitals' net margins slipped to 4.7 percent, the lowest level in five years, according to the latest annual performance data from the American Hospital Association (AHA 2000). Sagging finances were due to cutbacks in Medicare under the Balanced Budget Act, combined with managed care, losses from failed business strategies, and higher wage and pharmaceutical costs. Slumping prices in the stock market are exacerbating the problem, cutting into hospitals' investment income. Wall Street's Moody Investment Service predicts a long-term negative credit outlook for hospitals, as financial woes are translated into lower bond ratings.

E-solutions with payoff potential include electronic claims submission, billing software that optimizes charges, electronic charge capture systems, and managed care contract management systems. One-third of hospitals in a recent survey reported they were "using heavily" or "using satisfactorily" Internet connections with payers, and another 37 percent were planning to iniate Web connectivity with payers in the coming year (Morrisey 2001).

Benchmarking

America's best 100 hospitals are high-performing examples of superior management and high-quality medical outcomes. According to the latest ratings by Solucient, these top-ranked institutions consistently achieve shorter inpatient stays, lower costs per case, and superior clinical outcomes, despite treating more difficult cases (Solucient 2001).

Consultants estimate that total U.S. health costs would decline by $12 billion and 87,000 fewer deaths and 57,000 fewer complications would occur if all 5,000 hospitals could perform at the level of those ranked in the top 100. A growing number of hospitals and health systems are building dashboards of benchmarks and clinical indicators for medical staff, management, and the board. In San Diego, Sharp Health's senior vice president for clinical effectiveness, John Byrne, M.D., is leading a team to implement an outcome reporting system (Byrne 2001). The quarterly reports will focus on 33 disease states, which account for approximately 75 to 85 percent of the health system's patient volume.

Clinical Quality Improvement

Every hospital in the United States will pay closer attention to quality, and employers are backing electronic solutions for quality improvement. The Leapfrog Group, a coalition of 60 major employers, launched a nationwide initiative in late 2000. The employers promise to move their employees to hospitals that perform the best in treating patients (*New York Times* 2000). The employers in the coalition, including General Motors, IBM, and AT&T, will survey hospitals on whether they engage in three proven safety programs:

- electronic order-entry systems that ensure prescription drug orders are matched to patient and condition;
- use of intensivists to supervise intensive care units; and
- adherence to recommended guidelines for number of heart patients who are treated with coronary bypass procedures.

Care Management

The science of care management has been translated into care management protocols and electronic data analysis. Marshall Ruffin, M.D., a medical informatics consultant, argues that the real definition of an "integrated care system" includes the ability to share information according to a standard set of definitions and manage care consistently within organizationwide algorithms (Ruffin 1999). This level of systemwide care integration is still far from the norm. More than 50 percent of hospitals responding to the 2001 *Modern Healthcare* survey have no plans to implement any Web-related efforts in the care management area (Morrisey 2001). The Leapfrog Group cites examples in which e-enabled care management systems are reducing costs while improving quality. In Baltimore, specialists from the Johns Hopkins University have developed an electronic ICU monitoring and telemedicine system that telemonitors ICU patients on a 24 × 7 basis (*Business Wire* 2000). Their company, VISICU, mounted a four-month study that showed a 60 percent reduction in severity-adjusted mortality, 40 percent fewer complications, a 30 percent decrease in length of stay, and a 28 percent reduction in cost per case. Aggressively implementing Leapfrog's quality solutions pays off, reports Boston-based Brigham and Women's Hospital, a multiyear winner of the coveted rating as one of the top 100 hospitals in the United States. The hospital reports that it invested $1.9 million to conform to Leapfrog standards and has profited handsomely, reaping annual savings of $5 to $10 million (Trustee 2001).

Reducing Variation

The use of benchmarks among the top 100 hospitals is providing momentum to e-based initiatives to reduce clinical variation in areas such as length of stay. Among the Solucient top 100 hospitals, length of stay averaged 4.1 days last year, 7 percent lower than the national average of 4.4 days. Longer inpatient stays and more intensive use of resources make a big difference in the financials. Cost per case among the top 100 was $3,509, based on comparisons using 1996 Medicare data, whereas the national discharge cost averaged $4,365, or 24 percent higher (Solucient 2001). Benchmarking relies on an extensive internal database, translated into indicators which can be compared with best-practice benchmarks from the top 100, as well as with benchmarks from other reference bases. The Health Care Financing Administration hopes to widen the use of benchmarking among U.S. hospitals to reduce variance in clinical outcomes. HCFA recently released 24 process-of-care measures relating to prevention and treatment of six high-volume medical conditions, including heart attack, breast cancer, diabetes, congestive heart failure, peneumonia, and stroke (Allan 2000). Current Medicare data indicate substantial differences by region in clinical outcomes and the quality of care. This project is the first stage of a $240 million, three-year effort by HCFA to improve the quality of seniors' healthcare.

Physician Networks

Linking physicians in hospital-sponsored intranets will be one of the most effective strategies for physician alignment in the post-acquisition era. Two of three U.S. hospitals are currently working to provide Web access to its medical staff (Morrisey 2001). The Internet is

Figure 12.2: Physicians Online

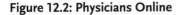

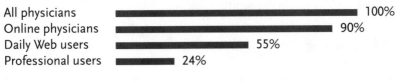

All physicians   100%
Online physicians   90%
Daily Web users   55%
Professional users   24%

Source: Hoppszallern (2001, p. 53).

simplifying the costs of connecting doctors with their hospitals. Doctors are showing more interest in computer linkages, as more physicians become regular Internet users. According to a national survey by Deloitte Research and Cyber Dialogue, 90 percent of doctors have accessed the Internet at some time in the past year (Hoppszallern 2001). More than half (55 percent) of practicing physicians are daily users, although the proportion of doctors using the Web for professional activities is still low, at 24 percent (see Figure 12.2).

Reducing Medical Errors

The Institute of Medicine's latest report on medical errors, *Crossing the Quality Chasm,* characterizes the current health system as "plagued by a serious quality gap" and calls for the end of handwritten clinical information by the year 2010 (Lovern 2001). IOM recommends that Congress create a $1 billion "innovation fund" for R&D in error reduction and clinical quality improvement. Although the Institute of Medicine is not a regulatory agency, physicians and hospitals fear the IOM report will lead to future government regulation. The price tag for upgrading the nation's healthcare information systems was not estimated by the Institute of Medicine but would certainly be in the billions of dollars. Providers see the demand for accountability on medical errors as another potential "unfounded mandate," and the American Hospital

Association's senior vice president, Carmela Coyle, remarked that, "funding is clearly going to be critical to bring about the kind of change that the IOM is talking about."

E-Reengineering

The focus on costs in health organizations is leading to renewed initiatives in reengineering and process improvement. Capital investments in electronic medical records will pay off because they address one of the greatest inefficiencies in healthcare—the immobility of medical records. The health system has always moved the *patient* rather than the *information* from location to location (Friend 2000). In addition, one in four hospitals is engaged in improving physician workflow, according to a recent *Modern Healthcare* survey (Morrisey 2001). Management consultant Michael Hammer, whose books on reengineering launched a global management movement in the 1990s, is pleased that the e-revolution is reenergizing his ideas on remaking organizations. Hammer argued in *Re-Engineering the Corporation* and in several follow-up management texts that companies should tear down their hierarchical structures and completely redesign their operations around key processes. This second wave of reengineering relies on electronic solutions and the Internet to take costs out of core processes such as inventory management, supply-chain management, and business-to-business transactions. Hammer has some advice for those suffering from "change fatigue" and are not eager for another wave of reengineering: "Suck it up. Live with it. Get used to it. In other words, no whining" (Church 1999, p. 3).

E-Recruitment

Internet access and interactive web sites are providing some solutions to healthcare's staffing crisis. Across the nation, more than 100,000 nursing vacancies are the symptom of a major national problem in finding staff for hospitals, medical offices, home health, laboratories, long-term care, and physical therapy. Virtually every provider is coping with staffing shortages, dwindling numbers of students emerging from the training pipeline, and wage wars, which only drive up costs without producing additional workers. Use of online recruitment is increasing rapidly among healthcare organizations. A recent survey by the Health Information Management Systems Society reported that 70 percent of hospital web sites provided recruitment information (IHC 2000). Most hospital web sites offering job listings also allow online submission of resumes and employment applications. The speed of the Internet enables a job seeker to send a resume and receive an acknowledgment in hours, rather than days or weeks. Telephone calls to job seekers are also reduced, with acknowledgment of resumes sent via the Web and job offers sent via e-mail.

Outsourcing

Outsourcing is one of the hottest trends in e-business. It is a highly flexible approach in which IT services and technology are available on a bundled or unbundled basis; vendors offer turn-key services or partial outsourcing arrangements for specific technologies, staffing, service and maintenance, or management activities. Healthcare organizations can turn over IT operations to a single contractor which may, in turn, subcontract with multiple firms. At the JPS Health Network, part of the Tarrant County Hospital District in Fort Worth, Texas, Info-Health Management has the master contractor relationship with JPS but employs several other companies for specific functions, such as hardware and software installation, network security, managing the web site, and providing a help desk (Pasternak 2001).

Performance incentives can be built into the outsourcing contract. St. Vincent Hospital and Health System in Indianapolis has an outsourcing arrangement with Daou, an IT outsourcing firm in San Diego, which includes 20 indicators that measure achievement of the IT system's goals and user satisfaction. To be compensated at the top of the fee range, Daou must reach the top level of performance as prescribed by the agreement. Outsourcing can also be the solution for HIPAA, which has a two-year timetable for compliance. Many hospitals may outsource their HIPAA activities rather than hire and train additional staff.

LOOKING FORWARD: THE E-CULTURE CHALLENGE

Information systems are considered the "spinal cord" of integrated healthcare organizations. New research findings on healthcare integration by Dean Coddington, Kenneth Ackerman, and Keith Moore of the McManis Consulting firm suggest that IDNs must do more than invest heavily in information technology: "It is necessary to invest smart (pick the right investments, in the right sequence) and to leverage the investments by building the support and culture to take full advantage of them" (Coddington, Ackerman, and Moore 2001, p. 3).

As the digital transformation occurs within the health sector, every hospital, medical group, health plan, and supplier must face the electronic-culture challenge to prepare themselves for the move to an e-based set of internal processes and external relationships. Healthcare organizations that grew by horizontal and vertical integration in the competitive 1970s and 1980s often see the small-scale, highly flexible e-organization model as a threat. Critics of struggling e-health companies like PlanetRx, drkoop.com and WebMD have correctly noted that some Internet businesses have lost investor confidence due to the lack of fundamental old-economy management practices, like growing revenues and making profits.

Canadian e-business consultant Karl Moore highlights six key factors in making a successful e-culture transition (Moore 2000).

1. Operate at Net speed—In an electronic marketplace, things are done much faster than in traditional firms. The ability to be nimble, innovative, and responsive to the market quickly are capabilities that large, traditional firms typically cannot match.
2. Execute dynamic strategy—Responsiveness is the hallmark of an e-culture, which accepts the need to make fast changes and is willing to build and launch new business models on a regular basis.
3. Have global reach—The world is the market, subject only to the boundaries of language, culture, and brands. E-culture

emphasizes worldwide learning, customer segments in many countries, and 24 × 7 service.

4. Enable e-initiatives—Across the organization, there must be many technology enthusiasts who will champion e-initiatives. "Moore's Law" of the expanding potential of information technology dictates new possibilities will appear every 18 to 24 months (Evans and Wurster 2000).

5. Engage in internal collaboration—Cutting across traditional silos of the organization, multifunctional teams come together around a goal and disband just as quickly to work on new goals.

6. Integrate with partners—In the new economy, no one firm can do it all. Working well with others is a fundamentally important skill.

Despite all the attention focused on e-business, management consultants say the skills needed to win in the digital economy are many of the same skills that have always been necessary for success, according to a recent survey by A. T. Kearney's executive search subsidiary (McDonald and Kallile 2000). At the end of the day, healthcare is still a local business with a risk-averse culture that is not an early adopter of technology. The dot-coms challenged the fundamentals of running a successful business, and they seem to have lost. The rules of operating any enterprise have not changed: having capital, systems, and experienced management is still essential. To be a high-performance organization, add vision, leadership, and culture.

Recognize that the e-revolution is not coming to the health field; it is already here. Every healthcare enterprise is currently straddling the digital divide. In the very near future, demanding patients will want access to their electronic medical records on the same basis as a doctor or nurse. Health plans will only pay electronic claims. Government will regulate medical errors, with mandatory electronic reporting. Employers will insist on accountability for costs and quality, with electronic report card ratings on every provider and plan. The supply chain will be 90 percent automated. The digital transformation of healthcare is only one way to meet these future market requirements.

STRATEGIC IMPLICATIONS

As technology becomes increasingly sophisticated, the so-called "soft side" of business, involving people and their motivations, turns out to matter more than ever (Pottruck and Pearce 2000). Innovation springs from the minds of people. Companies that understand the value alignment between individuals and the corporate culture can innovate at a faster rate. The kind of risk taking by individuals that is common in Internet-based enterprises must be supported by the organization's culture.

Transform at "Healthcare Speed." The digital transformation of healthcare will not take place at Internet speed. Most healthcare organizations cannot adapt that quickly. Some innovators and early adopters will outpace the industry, but most healthcare organizations will feel more comfortable being just a step or two behind.

Promote Change in the Middle of the Organization. Senior healthcare executives should understand that their middle managers must overcome two significant hurdles: they start with only limited understanding of the underlying technologies, and they have very limited slack time and resources to transition from old to new models. Time, training, technical assistance, and testimonials from other healthcare organizations will help hospitals and health systems move up the e-learning curve.

Be Patient. The digital transformation of healthcare will not take place overnight. The CIO of the Carle Clinic in Indiana recently exclaimed, "How can we afford to have both an EMR and a paper system; this is the worst of both worlds. We need to throw the paper away" (Coddington, Ackerman, and Moore 2001, p. 3). His frustration is natural. Be patient, and do not expect immediate progress or results. Despite the rhetoric of the e-revolution, expect at least a ten-year process of e-evolution.

REFERENCES

Allan, C. 2000. "Medicare Offers Quality Benchmarks." *On Managed Care* 5 (12): 5.

American Hospital Association (AHA). 2000. "Hospital Statistics 2001." Cited in "Hospital Vital Signs Lagging" by M. Mucklo. *On Managed Care* 6 (3): 1–2.

Barger, C. 2000. "IBM Transforms the Way People Work." [Online news story.] *Internet Wire*, December 18, p. 1.

Becker, C. 2001. "Checkmate: Computer 'Second Reads' of Mammograms Get a Lift from Congress." *Modern Healthcare* 31 (12): 62.

Business Wire. 2000. "VISICU Provides Solution to Leapfrog Group Healthcare Initiatives." [Online news story.] *Business Wire*, November 15, pp. 1–2.

Byrne, J. J. 2001. "A Revolutionary Advance in Disease Management." *Healthcare Leadership & Management Report* 9 (1): 14–20.

Church, E. 1999. "Hammer's Theory Hits on the Internet." [Online article.] *The Globe and Mail*, April 16, pp. 1–4.

Coddington, D. C., F. K. Ackerman, Jr., and K. D. Moore. 2001. "Integrated Health Care Systems: Major Issues and Lessons Learned." *Healthcare Leadership & Management Report* 9 (1): 1–9.

Coile, R. C., Jr. 1999. *Millennium Management: Better, Faster, Cheaper Strategies for Managing 21st Century Healthcare Organizations*. Chicago: Health Administration Press.

Eisinger, J. 2000. "Aiming in a New Direction." [Online article.] *Association Management*, April, pp. 1–3. Washington, DC: American Society of Association Executives.

Evans, P., and T. S. Wurster. 2000. *Blown to Bits: How the New Economy of Information Transforms Strategy*. Cambridge, MA: Harvard Business School Press.

Flory, J. 2001. "Washington State System Finds Web Success Through Vendor Relationship." *Internet Healthcare Strategies* 3 (3): 1–4.

Friend, D. B. 2000. *HealthCare.com: Rx for Reform*. Boca Raton, FL: St. Lucie Press.

Gartner's Business Technology Journal. 2000. "E-Enterprise: The Launch Pad for Innovation and Profit in the Digital Economy." Gartner Administrative Application Strategies Research Note, DF-12-5721, November 29. Cited in *The View from the Bridge*. Cambridge, MA: C-Bridge.

Goldsmith, J. 2001. "How Hospitals Should Be Using the Internet." *COR Healthcare Market Strategist* 2 (1): 1, 15–18.

Health Care Advisory Board Daily Briefing. 2001. "Sherman: Illinois Hospital Co-Pilots Ambulance Camera Program." [Online news brief.] News Tidbits, p. 2. Southfield, MI: Superior Consultant.

Hoppszallern, S. 2001. "Physicians and the Internet." *Hospitals & Health Networks* 75 (2): 51–55.

Inside Healthcare Computing (IHC). 2000. "Hospitals Are Pleased with Own Web Site Efforts: Many Spend Little." *Inside Healthcare Computing* 10 (11): 7–8.

Institute of Management and Administration (IOMA). 2000. "How Will E-Business Affect Your Company, and What Should You Do Now to Get Ready?" [Online article.] *Managing the General Ledger,* May 1, pp. 1–3.

Internet Wire. 2001. "BaseSix Business Model Produces Balance, Results for Growing Companies." [Online news story.] *Internet Wire,* March 6, pp. 1–2.

Lovern, E. 2001. "IOM Strikes Again." *Modern Healthcare* 31 (10): 4–6.

McDonald, D., and C. Kallile. 2000. "Digital Economy May Change, But Attributes of Leaders Don't, According to Kearney Survey." [Online news story.] *PR Newswire,* November 8, pp. 1–4.

McGowan, J. J. 2000. "Energy Management.com: How Will the Internet Change this Industry?" [Online article.] *Energy User News,* July 1, pp. 1–8.

Moore, K. 2000. "The E-volving Organization." [Online article.] *Ivey Business Journal,* November 1, pp. 25–28.

Morrisey, J. 2001. "Wanting More from Information Technology." Modern *Healthcare* 31 (6): 66–84.

Mucklo, M. 2001. "The Future of Medication Dispensing?" *On Managed Care* 6 (3): 7.

New York Times. 2000. "Naming Hospitals, Good and Bad." [Online news story.] *New York Times,* November 17, p. 34.

Pasternak, A. 2001. "Variations in Outsourcing: What's Right for You?" *Modern Healthcare,* Eye on Info (Suppl.): 6, 23.

Pottruck, D. S., and T. Pearce. 2000. *Clicks and Mortar: Passion-Driven Growth in an Internet-Driven World.* San Francisco: Jossey-Bass.

PR Newswire. 2000. "New Advanced Features Offer Anytime Flexibility for Small Businesses and Organizations." [Online news story.] *PR Newswire,* November 6, pp. 1–2.

Reeder, L. 2001. "Healthcare Industry Turning to E-Business Technologies Despite Obstacles, According to CSC Survey." *Healthcare Leadership & Management Report* 9 (1): 23–24.

Ruffin, M. D., Jr. 1999. *Digital Doctors.* Tampa, FL: American College of Physician Executives.

Schwartz, J. 2001. "Business on Internet Time." *New York Times,* March 30, pp. C1–C2.

Solovy, A. 2000. "Health Care's Most Wired: Is an E-Commerce Gap Emerging Among the Nation's Hospitals?" *Hospitals & Health Networks* 74 (4): 30–41.

Solucient. 2001. "100 Top Hospitals: Benchmarks for Success." Cited in "Hospital Vital Signs Lagging," by M. Mucklo. *On Managed Care* 6 (3): 1–2.

Trustee. 2001. "Taking Initiative on Medical Errors." [Online news story.] *Dow Jones Interactive,* January 1, p. 1.

Wall Street Journal. 2001. "HealthSouth, Oracle to Announce Joint Effort for 'Digital Hospital'." [Online news brief.] News Tidbits, March 26. pp. 1–2. Southfield, MI: Superior Consultant.

About the Author

Russell C. Coile, Jr., m.b.a., is National Strategy Advisor of Superior Consultant Company, a national consulting firm based in Southfield, Michigan, which provides digital business transformation services to more than 2,000 clients in the health field. He provides market forecasts and strategic advice to hospitals, medical groups, health plans, and suppliers on a nationwide basis.

Russ Coile is the author of eight books and numerous articles published on the future of the health field in the past 15 years, including *Futurescan 2001*, an annual environmental trends report (January 2001). His latest book, *Russ Coile's Health Forecast*, was just released by Aspen Publishers in December 2000. His monthly newsletter, *Russ Coile's Health Trends*, is now in its 13th year. For the past ten years his annual "top ten" predictions for the health field have been 90 percent accurate.

In the past year he participated in more than 100 seminars for groups, including:

- American Hospital Association
- American College of Healthcare Executives
- The Governance Institute

- American College of Physician Executives
- Rand Healthcare Roundtables

He is the past president of the Society for Healthcare Strategy and Market Development of the American Hospital Association and a member of several editorial advisory boards, including *Managed Care Outlook, Healthcare System Strategy Report, Nurse Week, Medical Network Strategy Report,* and *Healthcare Strategist.* His new column, "Future Trends," is published bimonthly by the *Journal of Healthcare Management.*

Mr. Coile holds a B.A. from the Johns Hopkins University and an M.B.A. in Health Services Administration from the George Washington University. His office is based in Plano, Texas.

He speaks to a wide variety of audiences on topics including:

- New Strategies for American Healthcare in the 21st Century
- Futurescan 2001: Millennium Forecast of Trends 2001–2005
- Millennium Management: "Better, Faster, Cheaper Strategies" for Healthcare
- Tracking the Trends: Evaluating Ten Years of Healthcare Forecasts
- E-Health: The Digital Transformation of Healthcare
- Beyond Managed Care: Reinventing the Industry on a Collaborative Model
- Techno-Medicine: Healthcare's New Frontier
- Physicians in Management: A Health Systems Perspective
- Rural Health: Challenges and Strategies

Mr. Coile is based in Washington, TX. He may be contacted at Russell_Coile@superiorconsultant.com.

Index

APQC. *See* American Productivity and Quality Center
Artificial intelligence, 194, 289
Ask a Nurse, 66, 177
Assessment tools, 17
Asymmetric digital subscriber loop (ADSL), 36
At-risk outsourcing arrangements, 43
Automated call distributor (ACD), 192
Automated decentralized pharmacy dispensing system (ADPDS), 30
Automated medication distribution systems, 288–89
Automated systems, 29–30

Baby boom generation, 57–58
Balanced Budget Act (BBA), 15, 17, 82, 219
Bandwidth, 212–13
Benchmark, 67, 74, **245**, 294
Benefits Improvement and Protection Act, 220
BHCAG. *See* Buyers Health Care Action Group
Blue Cross–Blue Shield Association, 15
Blue Cross of California, 114
Borgess Medical Center, 239
Brand identity, 5, 144–45
Bridge Medical, 230, 288
Brigham and Women's Hospital, 145, 295–96
Broadlane, 94
Browser limitations, 109
BSP. *See* Business service provider
Business processes, *xix*
Business service provider (BSP), 83, 164
Business-to-business (B2B), 20, 77, 78
  e-commerce, 5–6
  e-health strategies, 86–98
  evaluation, 101
  exchange, 85–86, 90–92
  in healthcare, 80–82, **83**
  online medical buying, 92–93
  pricing models, 83
Business-to-consumer (B2C), 4–5, 20, 80
Buyers Health Care Action Group (BHCAG), 179

CAD. *See* Computer assisted detection system
CaduCIS. *See* Clinical and Administrative Decision-Support Utility and Clinical Information System
CAHPS. *See* Consumer Assessment of Health Plans
California Healthcare Foundation, 163
Call center, *xx* , 66, 177
  alternative medicine information, 191
  components, 191–95
  cost-benefit analysis, 184–86
  costs, 191, **192**
  customer service, 188
  disease management application, 183
  as emergency hot lines, 188–89
  expenditures on, 178
  functions, 179
  guidelines, 184
  health promotion, 191
  interactive voice response system, 86–88
  issues, 180–82, **181**
  managed care and, 182–83
  mass customization, 190–91
  preventive medicine and, 189–90
  sponsors, 178
  staff-centered, 195–96
  vision, 190
  volume, 178
Capitated consulting, 43
Cardinal Health, 96, 99–100
Care Data Exchange, 163, 240–41
Care management
  algorithms, 183–84
  cost savings, *xv*, 106–7
  digital strategies, 295–96
  electronic solutions, 115–16
  software program, 229
CareScience, 229, 239, 240–41
CareTech Solutions, 159, 165
Case management, 10
Cash flow, 30
Catholic Healthcare West, 135, 243–44
Cedars-Sinai, 42
Celebrities, 136
Cellular phones, 45
Center Core, 181

Center for Patient Safety, 228
ChainOnline, 96
Change, 109
Chat rooms, 9
Chief information officer (CIO), *xv*,
    162–63, **162**
Chief medical information officer
    (CMIO), 36
Chief medical officer (CMO), 36
Children's Hospital of Philadelphia,
    136–37
CHIM. *See* College of Healthcare
    Information Management
CHINS. *See* Community health
    information networks
CHMIS. *See* Community health
    management information system
Chronic illness, 39, 244–45
CIGNA, 15, 90
Cimtek Commerce, 92, 93
CIO. *See* Chief information officer
Cleveland (Ohio) Clinic, 11, 13
Clicks-and-bricks strategy, 3, 100–101
Clinical and Administrative
    Decision-Support Utility and
    Clinical Information System
    (CaduCIS), 229
Clinical collaboratives, 227
Clinical decision-making model, 234–36
Clinical indicators, 38
Clinical information system, 36
Clinical practice variations, 234–36
Clinical protocols, 16
Clinical trials, 10, 12, 16
CME. *See* Continuing medical education
CMIO. *See* Chief medical information
    officer
CMO. *See* Chief medical officer
Coding, 167–68
Collaborative commerce, 283, 287–88
Collections, 30
College of Healthcare Information
    Mangement (CHIM), 186
Communication, 191
Community education, 69–70
Community Health Care, 237
Community health information
    networks (CHINS), 63, 111, 163,
    268–69

Community health management
    information system (CHMIS), 63
Community service, 189
Comparative market data, 72–73
Computer assisted detection (CAD)
    system, 289
Computer service provider
    (CSP), 169
Computer telephony integration (CTI),
    191, 193
Connections, 206
Connectivity, 287–88
Consultation, 10, 26
Consumer
    confidence, 53–57
    control, 260
    education, 72
    empowerment, *xviii*, *xix–xx*, 131
    essential information, **71**
    expectations, 228
    focus groups, 66–67
    hot lines, 66
    information, 189
    informed, 73
    ratings, 59
    report card use, 70–73
    satisfaction, 52, 67–68
    surveys, 68
    telemedicine acceptance, 220
Consumer Assessment of Health Plans
    (CAHPS), 60
Consumerism, 49–50, 64
Continuing medical education (CME),
    30, 169
Co-opetition, 100, 168
Cost data, 29–30
Crisis centers, 136
CSP. *See* Computer service provider
CTI. *See* Computer telephony
    integration system
Customer-focused, 64–70
Customer loyalty, 5
Customer relationship management
    (CRM), 139–50, 161
Customer satisfaction, 73–74
Customer service, 14, 30
CVS, 13
Cyberchondriacs, 7
Cyber-marketing, 40–42

Electronic standards, 84, 109, 259
E-mail, 37
Emergency hot lines, 188–89
Emergency plan, 274
Emery University, 54
EmpactHealth.com, 94
Employee Benefit Research Institute
    (EBRI), 56–57
EMR. *See* Electronic medical record
Energy management, 30
Enrollment systems, 114
Enterprise application infrastructure, 35
Enterprise management, 29–30
Enterprise network, 63
Environmental services, 30
E-partnership, 291–92
E-recruitment, 298–99
E-reengineering, 298
Error reduction, 238–40
ESC. *See* Executive steering committee
Ethnic groups, 57
E-transactions, 113–14
Evanston Northwestern Healthcare, 42
Executive steering committee (ESC),
    162–63
Experts, 136
Expert systems, 194
Extensible markup language (XML),
    xvii, 214, 215
Extranet, 33, 37

False Claims Act, 265
Family Physicians of Northfield, 179
Finances, 19
Financial performance, 245–46, 293–94
First Consulting Group, 165
First Health, 210
Fisher Scientific, 99–100
Focus groups, 66–67
Foundation Health Systems, 90
Foundations, 13
Fundraising, 13

Gainsharing arrangement, 164
Gender gap, 57
Globalization, 301–2
Government protection issues, 254

Graphical user interface (GUI), 193
Group Health Cooperative of Puget
    Sound, 187
Group purchasing organization (GPO),
    83–84, 86, 93, 94

Hardware interoperability, 215
Hartford Foundation, 63
Harvard Pilgrim Health Care, 167
HCA Healthcare, 86, 94
HCFA. *See* Health Care Financing
    Administration
Healinx, 171–72
HealthAxis.com, 14, 84
Health benefit management consult-
    ants, 290
HealthBridge, 168
Healthcare
    delivery, 7
    digital strategies, 292–99
    e-commerce applications, **6**
    guides, 50–52
    integration strategies, 85
    Internet effect on, 82–84
    national extranet, 33
    technology applications, 288–89
    transaction costs, 5–6
Health Care Financing Administration
    (HCFA), 15, 61, 63
HealthCentral, 3, 98, 135
Health.com, 86
Health Data Management, 35, 36
Health data networks, 63
Healtheon Corporation, 7, 78–79,
    88, 90
HealthGate, 169
HealthGrades.com, 11, 51, 58, 145–46
Health and Human Services,
    Department of, 138, 228
Health information
    access to, *xvi*, 5
    availability of, *xix–xx*, 128
    consumer choices for, 8–10
    content provider, 134–35, 141–42
    disease-specific, 140–41
    interactive sites, 142–43
    library, 186
    online, 107, **107**, 127–28